MW00811375

INTERMITTENT FASTING FOR WOMEN OVER 50

The Easier Guide to Master The Secrets of Losing Weight.
Detoxify The Body and Gain Energy to Promote Longevity!

SYDNIE AMBERLY

TABLE OF CONTENTS

Introduction

Congratulations on purchasing
Intermittent Fasting for Women Over 50:
The Easier Guide to Master The Secrets of Losing Weight.
Detoxify The Body and Gain Energy to Promote Longevity!
And thank you for doing so.

The chapters in this book will be discussing each and every segment of intermittent fasting, specifically with respect to all women over the age of 50. Intermittent fasting has turned out to be quite famous in recent years, and it has also proven itself to be a very useful method for losing weight. Unlike other types of diets, intermittent fasting has nothing to do with the types of food that you consume. It is all about timing all your meals. You will find several other books on intermittent fasting that are written in a generalized format. This book brings up a comprehensive solution for all women over the age of 50 with respect to intermittent fasting. You will also find plenty of nutritional information within this book.

Many of you might think what exactly the difference is in intermittent fasting between men and women. Well, there are several differences as the nutritional requirements for women are not the same as men. Also, the body of women works in a different way than men. So, this book is all about intermittent fasting is respect to women.

There are several books available in the market today on Intermittent Fasting. Every effort has been made to make this book as interesting as possible. Enjoy!

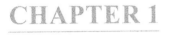

CHAPTER 1

WHAT IS
INTERMITTENT
FASTING?

There is nothing new and fancy about fasting. It has been coming along since the ancient years. However, there are various individuals who just try to brush it away as a mere rule of society without backing it up with any kind of scientific benefit or explanation. But, if you try to study it a bit, you will very easily come to know about the various benefits of intermittent fasting and how beneficial it is for your body. By gaining knowledge about fasting, more people are attentive to the various benefits of fasting. Intermittent fasting is also a type of fasting where the fast is maintained according to a specific timetable or routine. You will also find various cultures and religions all over the world that lays stress on the importance and requirement of fasting.

You will also come to know about various medical surgeries or even tests that come with the requirement of fasting. But, when it comes to the benefits of fasting with respect to weight loss, it is not that common among the people in spite of the fact that there various theories for backing up the claim. In several cases, people even take fasting to be a very unhealthy practice. But, is fasting really unhealthy in nature?

Well, the answer to this very question relies on the way in which you practice fasting. If you are into intermittent fasting, then it cannot be considered as unhealthy when you have a clear idea of how to carry on with it by following the rules. Your body will enter the state of fasting but unlike normal fasting, each and every necessary nutrient that is required for maintaining all the beneficial functions of the body will be present. You are also required to remember that losing weight because of intermittent fasting is not at all a negative result but a positive one.

There are also various individuals who just confuse regular diet plans with intermittent fasting. But intermittent fasting has no relation to the normal diets. The most common diet plans that are being followed by people are based on limiting their calorie intake and altering the macronutrient type that they take in one day. But when it comes to intermittent fasting, it is focused on the eating time and then starting the required changes and effects in the body. You will be following a specific pattern of diet that comes with various eating phases and wit fasting, where both are altered with one another. When you are in the stage of fasting while practicing intermittent fasting, you will be restricted from having any kind of food that can readily add up to the calorie count. You can drink or eat only during the eating phase. In this phase, you can consume all those food items that come with a certain value of calories.

A very common belief among most people is that when someone practices intermittent fasting, it is enough for inducing loss of weight all alone. But in actuality; it is not the case. Weight loss takes place because of calorie deficiency and that is why you are required to limit the number of meals that you have as this will only limit your total eating time. But, when it comes to intermittent fasting, it does not only rely on the calorie content or value of calories in one whole day. This form of fasting is much more sustainable in nature when compared to other diet forms. It is very flexible in nature and can bring in greater satisfaction levels when it comes to the concept of fasting.

The simplicity that is associated with the overall process of intermittent fasting is that it is more concerned about the time when you are consuming food and not really about what you are consuming. You can rid yourself of the daily hassle of properly counting all the calories each and every time when you cook any snacks or meals for yourself. The choices of your food will be the same as it is and there is no need for restricting yourself from consuming all the tasty dishes that are generally limited by the other forms of diets. The best part, you are not required to strictly follow any kind of meal plan every day as intermittent fasting is not concerned about any fixed portion of micronutrients.

Intermittent Fasting And The Various Myths

Intermittent fasting has turned out to be immensely popular today and there is no doubt that is it one of the trending topics in the fitness world. Most of us have read about it on social media or have heard about the same from any friend. But, it is a common thing to see that whenever any new concept comes up, there has to be some kind of myths associated with it. For debunking all those myths, you are required to dive in deeper and find out the actual scenario. Here are some of the most commonly heard misconceptions about intermittent fasting that are needed to be cleared before starting with intermittent fasting.

Intermittent Fasting Is A Starvation Diet

This can be regarded as the biggest of all the myths. Fasting is not going to put your body in shut down mode. If you just skip any meal or two or even try fasting for one whole day, you will not be starving. Based on several pieces of research, for the rate of metabolism of your body to drop down, you will need to fast for a period of 60 hours straight. You need to understand that the human body has been designed in such a way that it can very easily tackle all the hours of fasting without even giving in or falling down. According to a study from the American Journal of Physiology, fasting for a period of 36 to 48 hours can increase the rate of metabolism from 3.5% straight to 10%.

One thing that needs to be cleared is that starving and fasting are completely different concepts. While starving, the human body enters in an extreme condition, which might even result in death because of excessive hunger. At the time of starving, the deposits of fat in the body start to deplete and thus, the muscles in the body start breaking down for filling up the requirements of energy for the body. While practicing intermittent fasting, it is only the deposits of fat that get affected, which are broken down for the purpose of releasing the required energy. In intermittent fasting, there is no form of damage in the body muscles and lean tissues. Intermittent fasting will not be harming unless and until the body fat percentage tends to go below 5% and the individual keeps himself/herself busy in various types of physical activities. Always keep one thing in mind, carry on with intermittent fasting in the proper way and if required under proper guidance or supervision.

In intermittent fasting, there is no chance of starving yourself as intermittent fasting is all about alternate phases of eating and fasting. You will be following one fixed pattern.

Intermittent Fasting Can Make You Feel Hungry For The Whole Day

It has been found from various researches that as you fast, your hunger level will also be decreasing. For instance, when an individual who is suffering from obesity enters the second week of their intermittent fasting schedule, they will not be feeling hungry like before and their hunger level will also be low. It has also been found that it is tougher to properly maintain the intake of calories during the days of fasting than having control over your hunger.

Consuming More Meals Can Easily Boost Up The Rate Of Metabolism

You must have come across various individuals in your life who just wants to eat more only because they want to prevent their metabolic rate from falling down. They have the notion that as you have more meals, you are burning down more calories. There is a very famous term which is known as the TEF or thermic effect of food. The TEF can define the total number of calories that are being burnt right after having a meal. Generally, the value of TEF corresponds to 10% of the total number of calories that are being consumed.

So, it can be stated that it is not at all important how frequently you had your meals but what your total intake of calories is. If you are having a total of 3 meals of 1000 calories and someone else is consuming six meals of 500 calories, the overall effect will be the same. In both cases, the value of TEF is 10%, which will be amounting to 3000 calories. The overall number of calories that our body burns in one day would not be affected even if we increase or decrease the meal frequency.

Your Level Of Hunger Will Be Reduced If You Have Frequent Meals

This is another myth that we all believed at some point in time in our lives. Many people believe that the easiest way of dealing with excessive cravings and hunger is by engaging in a periodic form of eating. A research was conducted on the effects of protein intake and was performed with a comparison between consuming 6 high-protein meals in one day and having 3 high-protein meals in the course of the day. The result concluded that it is enough to have three meals for dealing with hunger.

However, you will be coming across various types of evidence in regard to this point. This is because the food responses will vary from person to person and it will also depend on the requirements of nutrition by the individual.

You Will Start Losing Muscles Once You Start With Intermittent Fasting

You will come across various people who will be telling you not to start with intermittent fasting as it might lead to the reduction of body muscles. But in actuality, it is not at all true. There are several reports where bodybuilders used intermittent fasting for increasing their muscle mass and for eliminating all forms of body fat. So, there is no form of evidence that can support muscle loss resulting from intermittent fasting much more than in any other limitation in calories.

Anything Can Be Consumed In The Phase Of Eating

Even though we said that you will not need any kind of meal plan while intermittent fasting, that does not indicate that you can consume anything you want. Consuming everything and that too in large amounts can be regarded as one of the reasons why many people fail to continue to intermittent fasting. This is the very reason why most people find it tough to keep up with the goals that they fix up, followed by disappointment as they fail in achieving all those goals. It is true that you have kept up with the fast for a long period of time. But, that does not mean you can consume anything you want to in the eating phase.

Your body burns a fixed amount of calories every day based on all your features and the total amount of work that you perform in one day. If you have the notion that consuming more calories in the phase of eating than the amount that is being burnt will not be affecting your body and health in any possible way, then you are absolutely wrong. It will possibly be increasing your body weight and thus making you obese. Losing weight is always the result of a calorie deficit that you can create in your diet. Also, maintaining a properly balanced diet will make it easier for you to keep a count on your calories. You need to avoid all those food items that are high in preservatives such as canned or processed foods. You can opt for whole food items that are fresh and rich in nutrients as well.

CHAPTER 2

WHAT ARE THE BENEFITS AND RISKS OF INTERMITTENT FASTING?

Intermittent fasting comes along with a wide array of benefits along with some risks as well. Everything in this world comes with a bad and a good side and so does intermittent fasting. Let's have a look at them.

Benefits

Intermittent fasting has been gaining its popularity in regard to the various types of benefits that it imparts on our health and body. It has been found from various studies that intermittent fasting can have some powerful types of benefits on our brain and body. So, let's have a look at some of the benefits of this popular form of fasting.

Helps In Losing Belly Fat And Weight

Most of the people who opt for intermittent fasting are because of its immense results in weight loss. Intermittent fasting will allow you to eat a limited number of meals. Unless you just try to compensate by consuming more meals, you will be taking in fewer calories. In addition, intermittent fasting helps in enhancing the functions of various hormones for facilitating weight loss. Lower levels of insulin, increased amount of noradrenaline, and a higher level of growth hormone improves the breaking down of body fat and uses it up as the energy. For this very reason, fasting for short periods helps in increasing the rate of metabolism by 3.5% - 14% and thus helping you to burn more calories. Intermittent fasting actually works equally on both sides of the equation of calories. It helps in boosting up the rate of metabolism and reduces the total amount of food that we eat.

According to research from the year 2014, it has been

found that intermittent fasting can help in losing weight of 3% - 8% over the course of 4 – 24 weeks. This is actually a great amount of fat loss. You can lose 5% - 7 % of your waist circumference and thus indicating loss of belly fat, the harmful nature of fat that stores up in our abdominal cavity and results in various types of diseases. Thus it can be concluded that intermittent fasting is a great tool for losing belly fat and body weight while boosting up your metabolism.

Alters The Functions Of Genes, Hormones, And Cells

When you stop eating for a while, there are several things that are happening inside your body. For instance, your body will start with the beneficial repairing processes of the cells and alter the levels of hormones for making the stored body fat much more accessible. Let's have a look at some of the changes that take place in our body as we fast:

Insulin: The level of insulin in the blood drops down that helps in the burning of fat.

Growth hormone: The level of growth hormone rises almost by 5%. Higher levels of growth hormone help in gaining muscles and also facilitate fat burning.

Gene expression: Some important changes take place in various molecules and genes which are related to protection from diseases and longevity.

Cell repair: The body starts with various important cell repair processes like cleaning out cell waste materials etc.

Thus it can be said that intermittent fasting induces the body to change various functioning and level of hormones for imparting improved rate of fat burning.

Reduces Resistance To Insulin And Lowers Down The Risk Of Type 2 Diabetes

Type 2 diabetes has turned out to become immensely common in recent years. The main feature of it is higher levels of blood sugar in regard to insulin resistance. Anything that can reduce resistance to insulin can help in lowering the levels of blood sugar and also provide protection against this form of diabetes. Luckily, intermittent fasting has shown some great results in insulin resistance that can provide an effective reduction in the levels of blood sugar. While practicing intermittent fasting, fasting blood sugar can be reduced by 4% - 6% while the level of fasting insulin can be reduced by 21% - 30%. Also, intermittent fasting can protect you from the damage of your kidney as it is the most common form of complication that can be linked to diabetes. This implies that practicing intermittent fasting by people who are at the risk of developing diabetes can be protected from the risks of it. But, the overall effect of intermittent fasting in regard to insulin resistance will depend on the gender and body features.

Reduces Oxidative Stress Along With Inflammation

Oxidative stress is often regarded as one step closer to various chronic diseases along with aging. It includes the unstable molecules known as free radicals that react with the other necessary body molecules such as DNA and protein and thus damages them. Intermittent fasting can help in dealing with oxidative stress. It also comes with the added advantage of reducing inflammation in our body.

Helps In Improving The Health Of The Heart

The current biggest killer in the world is heart diseases. There are various risk factors that can be associated with the risk of developing heart disease. Intermittent fasting can help in improving various risk factors along with LDL cholesterol, blood pressure, inflammatory markers, blood triglycerides, and levels of blood sugar. So, it can be concluded that intermittent fasting can help in dealing with various heart diseases and thus, improving the health of the heart.

Induces Several Processes Of Cell Repair

As you fast, the body cells start with a process of waste removal from the cells known as autophagy. This whole process involves breaking down of the cells and metabolizing of the dysfunctional and broken proteins that slowly builds up inside the body cells. Increase level of autophagy can help in providing protection against various types of diseases that also includes Alzheimer's disease and cancer.

Helps In Preventing Cancer

Cancer is a very common and deadly disease today that is generally characterized by uncontrollable cell growth. Intermittent fasting has shown some important effects on body metabolism that can help in reducing the overall risk of developing cancer. Although it still needs human studies, evidence from various animal studies shows that intermittent fasting can help in preventing cancer.

Beneficial For The Brain

Anything that is good for our body is also good for our brain. Intermittent fasting helps in improving several metabolic features that have been found to be beneficial for the health of our brain. This also involves reduced levels of oxidative stress, reduced levels of blood sugar, resistance to insulin, and reduced inflammation. Several studies have been conducted in rats that show intermittent fasting can help in improving the growth of brand new nerve cells, which will directly benefit the functioning of the brain. It also helps in increasing the brain hormone level known as BDNF or brain-derived neurotrophic factor. The deficiency of this brain hormone can result in depression, along with various other problems of the brain. Intermittent fasting might also protect the brain from damages that result from strokes.

Might Help In Preventing Alzheimer's Disease

Alzheimer's disease is the most common type of neurodegenerative disease in the world. There is still no treatment or cure for this disease and so preventing this disease from developing is actually very critical. A study with rats showed that intermittent fasting might reduce the severity of Alzheimer's disease or delay its onset. In a long series of reports from various case studies that included regular short-term fasts, it was found that the diet was able to improve the symptoms of the disease in nine out of ten patients. It has also been found that intermittent fasting might also protect against the onset of Parkinson's disease.

Lesser Stored Fat
As your body enters the phase of fasting, both glucose and glycogen tend to get depleted really fast. So, your body will slowly get accustomed to using the lower levels of insulin in relation to certain blood sugar levels. Such form of low requirement of insulin by the body enhances the body's sensitivity towards this hormone. This will increase the body efficiency for utilizing all the available glucose in a much better way of releasing energy.

More Amount Of Lean Muscles
One of the major drawbacks of most of the strategies related to weight loss is that besides losing fat, they also result in losing muscle mass. But, when it comes to intermittent fasting, it does not even affect the lean mass. Losing mass of the muscles is the worst thing that can take place. Intermittent fasting does not harm your body's metabolism while still losing bodyweight. So, it can be concluded that with intermittent fasting, you can lose weight while not losing your muscle mass.

Reduced Cravings
Are you really fed up with all the cravings that force you to give up on your plans? This is a very common problem which is faced by most of the people. This is mainly because of an increase in insulin levels. While practicing intermittent fasting, you can easily keep insulin sensitivity under your control. Once your body attains a fixed level, your body will not be producing any extra insulin. So, all the sugar cravings that you have will stop eventually. You will also be able to deal

with hunger in a better way as you keep on practicing intermittent fasting.

Risks
Intermittent fasting is taken to be a very beneficial practice when it comes to weight loss. It also provides a series of other benefits as well but along with that, it comes with certain risks that need to be studied properly. As everything in this world comes along with a downside, intermittent fasting comes with so. If you really want to practice intermittent fasting by seeing all its benefits, you need to be aware of its drawbacks as well. Here are some drawbacks that are associated with intermittent fasting.

Orthorexia
Intermittent fasting might lead to disordered behaviors of eating like orthorexia. It is an obsession with eating healthy or properly. The symptoms of this behavior involve the urge to talk to someone regarding your daily diet all the time along with being preoccupied with the thought of what to eat next. If you find out that your diet pattern has turned out to be inflexible to the extent that you always want to avoid any kind of social events, just stop with the process and look out for some other weight loss method.

Disrupted Sleep
Although it has been found that not consuming any kind of food right before bedtime can improve your sleeping ability, it has also been found out that practicing intermittent fasting can also disrupt your cycle of sleep. It affects your sleep by decreasing the total REM sleep.

REM sleep is essential for mood regulation, learning capacity, and memory.

Reduced Alertness
While it is true that practicing intermittent fasting can improve your alertness, when practiced for the long term, it can also reduce it. This is mainly because your body does not get the required amount of fuel. Thus, it turns out to be incapable of producing more energy in the long run. It can also result in dizziness, fatigue, and difficulty in developing concentration.

Increase In Guilt
As you break your fast or miss out the window of fasting either by eating late or early can result in feelings of shame or anxiety. You need to be very cautious of such feelings as it might indicate something bigger such as a disordered pattern of eating.

Increased Levels Of Cortisol
As fasting is more or less like stress on your body just like working out, it can readily increase the level of cortisol in the body. The level readily increases when you try to keep yourself away from food for a long period of time. An increase in the level of cortisol can increase stress in the body along with the storage of fat.

Higher Levels Of LDL
Intermittent fasting can readily increase the levels of LDL in the body, which has been found from research by the American Journal Of Physiology.
Although several pieces of research are still being conducted, the effects of intermittent fasting for the

long-term are still unknown. So, always keep in mind that if you are willing to incorporate intermittent fasting within your routine, make sure that you consult with your doctor or parents before opting for it. If you are sure about practicing it, note that there is always a healthy and safe way of doing so.

CHAPTER 3

TYPES OF INTERMITTENT FASTING

Intermittent fasting is now being practiced for many years because of its advantage in regard to weight loss and a healthy body. It is somewhat similar to the ancient style of fasting but only with a certain change in its pattern. Today, intermittent fasting can be practiced by using several methods. You can choose the one that suits you the best or the one with which you can carry forward easily. Let's have a look at the types of intermittent fasting.

16/8 Method

In this type of intermittent fasting, the overall consumption of food along with the intake of calorie-rich beverages is only allowed for a limited window of eight hours. You will be fasting for the rest of the sixteen hours. You can repeat this cycle as many times you want-one time in a week or twice every week to even every day, depending on your own preference. 16/8 method of intermittent fasting has reached new heights in popularity in the last few years, specifically among all those people who want to burn body fat and lose weight. Unlike the other types of diets, the 16/8 method is very much easy to follow as is does not come along with any type of fixed regulations and rules.

You can get real results and that too with the least amount of effort. It is taken as more flexible and less restrictive in nature when compared to other types of diet plans. The best thing about this type of intermittent fasting is that it can be incorporated very easily in your lifestyle without any kind of hassle. Additionally, the 16/8 method also helps in improving the control of blood sugar level, enhances longevity, and also boosts up the functioning of the brain. It is a very safe, sustainable and simple form of fasting. For starting with this, you need to pick up a window of eight hours and just limit the intake of food only to that frame of time. Most of the people practicing this type of intermittent fasting prefer to have all their meals between 1 p.m. and 8 p.m. So, you will be fasting overnight and then skip your breakfast the next day. You will still be able to have a balanced dinner and lunch in addition to some snacks all throughout the course of the day.

There are people who just decide to keep their eating phase between 10 a.m. and 6 p.m. so that they can have enough time to have a properly balanced breakfast at 10 a.m., a balanced lunch at noon along with a very light snack or early dinner around 6 p.m. just before starting with the fast again. The best way of finding the perfect time frame is by experimenting and then picking the time that fits the best with your schedule. No matter when you eat, it is always suggested to have various small-sized meals along with snacks that are spread out evenly throughout the day. This is mainly because of the fact that you will be able to stabilize the levels of blood sugar and also keep your hunger under absolute control. For maximizing the health benefits of this type of intermittent fasting, you will need to stick to only nutritious whole food items along with beverages in your phase of eating.

You can balance every meal that you have in your eating phase by including various types of whole food items like: **Vegetables:** Cucumber, broccoli, leafy green vegetables, cauliflower, tomato, etc.

Fruits: Berries, bananas, apples, pears, peaches, oranges, etc.
Healthy fats: Avocado, olive oil, etc.
Whole grains: Oats, barley, quinoa, buckwheat, etc.
Protein: Fish, meat, nuts, eggs, poultry, legumes, etc.

You can also include beverages that are free from calories such as unsweetened coffee and tea at the time of fasting. It will help you to keep yourself hydrated along with controlling your appetite.

But, in this method of intermittent fasting, there might be some drawbacks. As the eating window is only for eight hours, you might consume more food than usual during your phase of eating and this might lead to gain in weight, problems with the digestive system, and might also result in the development of unhealthy habits of eating. As you start with this practice, you might also face some negative effects such as weakness, hunger, and fatigue because of the restricted eating phase. Although the 16/8 method of intermittent fasting is generally taken to be safe for all adults, it is always better to consult with your doctor right before you start with the practice. Also, women who are thinking of conceiving or are pregnant or are breastfeeding cannot attempt for this.

5:2 Diet

This is a very popular method of intermittent fasting in which you are required to reduce your food consumption for two days a week. It is also known as fast diet. This eating pattern will permit you to consume food in a normal way for 5 days and then on any two days that you choose, you will be restricting your intake of calories. As no food items are off the limits, this type of intermittent fasting is very appealing to all those people who are willing to get into shape or improve their overall health. In this meal plan, there are no types of complex diet that you need to follow. This is very simple in nature where you are not even required to count your calorie intake. You will be eating normally for the majority of the week and then restrict your overall intake of calories for the rest of the two days.

On the days of your fasting, you will be reducing your intake of calories to 600 (men) and to 500 calories (women). During the rest of the week, you can carry on with your normal meals. You can actually eat whatever you feel like in this type of intermittent fasting. There is nothing like bad food or good food. But, regardless of this fact, you should always try to opt for nutritious food items. This type of intermittent fasting will work the best if you can fill it up with fruits, lean proteins, veggies, healthy fats, and whole grains. It is very important to include protein and healthy fats in your diet as they can provide your body and brain with all the energy that is needed. Food items that are high in fiber content like broccoli and carrots can help in making you feel full.

During 5 days of the week when you will be eating normally, you are not meant to consume more food than usual. If you think that eating more on the normal days for compensating the requirement of your fasting days can help, you are completely wrong. You might end up gaining more weight instead of losing. Try to keep the normal days as normal as possible and omit any kind of high-sugar and high-calorie food. On the days of fasting, you can experiment with the time for finding out what works best for your body and brain. Some individuals can function their best by having a small light breakfast while other people just prefer waiting for a long time for having the first meal.

Your aim should be to consume around 25% of your daily calorie intake. As you only have very limited calories for working with, you can try to evenly spread them all throughout your meal routine. For instance, if you need to intake 500 calories on the days of fasting, you can consume 200 calories at the time of breakfast, 100 calories at the time of lunch, and the rest 200 calories at the time of dinner. You can also divide your total calorie count of 500 as 250 for lunch and the rest 250 for dinner.

Do not opt for keeping your fasting days consecutive to one another. Try keeping a gap of one or two days in between. For example, you can keep Sunday, Tuesday, Wednesday, Friday, and Saturday as your normal days while fasting on Monday and Thursday. While fasting, you might also experience certain side effects such as irritability, fatigue, headache, sleepiness, nausea, weakness, and many others. Such side effects are very much normal in nature and generally get normalized as your body gets used to the pattern of fasting. If you feel yourself getting overwhelmed while practicing this routine try to drink water more often or you can also keep yourself busy with work.
Always remember, if your calorie count is around 2000, do not try to reduce it suddenly. Take it slow, reduce

around 500 calories in the first week and continue doing so until it reaches 500 calories in total in a day.

Eat Stop Eat

This method of intermittent fasting includes fasting for 24 hours for one day or two days a week. This type of intermittent fasting was popularized by Brad Pilon who is a fitness expert. This method includes fasting from dinner of day one to dinner of day two. This will amount to total fasting of 24 hours. For instance, if you have your dinner at 8 p.m. on Monday and just stop your consumption of food till 8 p.m. on Tuesday, you will complete a total 24 hours fast. If you want you can also start your fasting from breakfast or lunch of day one till breakfast or lunch of day two. The end result will still be the same. You can consume coffee, water or other beverages that have zero calories at the time of fasting but you cannot consume any kind of solid food before the 24 hours mark. If you are opting for this method of intermittent fasting for losing weight, it is of utter importance that you consume food normally during your days of eating.

But, this 24-hour fast might turn out to be actually difficult for many people. There is no need for rushing with it. You can start with your fast as 12 hours or 16 hours and gradually increase that time frame to 24 hours. The main benefit of this method is that there is no need to keep yourself hungry every day in a week. You can have anything you want during your periods of eating. You can fast for either one or two days, depending on your health and lifestyle.

The eat stop eat method is not at all a strict routine of

fasting. It is more or less like a philosophy that only focuses on certain breaks from your eating routine. But, right before you start with this, make sure to identify your goals, needs, and abilities. Do not try to push it hard as it might hamper your health.

Alternate Day Fasting

The basic idea of this form of fasting is that you need to fast on day one and then eat again the next day. This way you can carry on with it with alternate days of fasting and eating. In alternate day fasting, you are only required to restrict what you consume half of the time. On the days of fasting, you can easily drink as many calorie-free beverages you want to such as tea, unsweetened coffee, and water. While following this method, you can only have about 500 calories on your days of fasting or about 25% of the total requirements of energy. The benefits of weight loss will still be the same if the calories of fasting days are consumed at the time of dinner or lunch or as several small-sized meals during the course of the day. It has been found that people often find it much easier to carry on with this method rather than the normal method of restricting calorie intake.

While following alternate day fasting, you can easily lose about 4% - 8% of your total body weight in about 3 – 12 weeks. It can also reduce the harmful belly fat along with inflammations in the body. Other than weight loss, this method also helps in dealing with type 2 diabetes. It can also reduce the levels of insulin in the body along with resistance to insulin. Alternate day fasting also helps in improving your heart health by reducing the circumference of your waist by decreasing your blood pressure and also by lowering the level of bad cholesterol or LDL by 25% in the body. On the days of fasting, you can consume food items such as berries with yogurt, veggies and eggs, salad along with lean meat, and others.

Warrior Diet

In this method of intermittent fasting, you need to consume veggies and fruits in small amounts during the day and then consume one large meal at your dinner. The basic idea is to fast for the whole day and then consume food at night within an eating window of four hours. During the fasting period of 20 hours, you can also consume light dairy products and eggs. You can have anything you want within the eating window at night but it is always recommended to opt for healthy and nutritious food items. It has been found that the warrior diet might help in losing weight. But, many people might end up consuming more than their normal calorie count at the time of eating as they fast throughout the day. So, you will need to keep a check on what you eat and drink in that eating period.

This method intermittent fasting also helps in reducing inflammation which is the key to various chronic diseases such as cancer, diabetes, heart diseases. But, it is not at all recommended for children under the age of 15, people who practice sports or athletes, people who suffer from being underweight, and pregnant women. It might often lead to anxiety and irritability, but you will get used to it with time.

Spontaneous Meal Skipping

In this method, you are not needed to follow any kind of fixed plan of intermittent fasting for reaping all the benefits of this method. This method of intermittent fasting, you just need to simply skip some of your meals with time, for example, at a time when you do not want to eat or you are very much busy with work for cooking and then eating. It is actually a myth that human beings need to eat after every few hours for not reaching the mode of starvation or for preventing loss of muscles which has already been discussed in the previous chapters. Your body is equipped properly for handling long periods of fast, so there is no harm in missing some of your meals in a day.

So, if you are not actually hungry or do not have the urge to eat, you can skip your breakfast one day and just have a complete dinner or lunch. If you are driving for long distances or traveling for a long time and you are unable to find something to eat, you can do a very short fast. You just need to ensure that you are having only healthy foods while consuming whole meals.

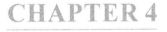

CHAPTER 4

WHAT TO EAT
AND WHAT
TO DRINK

Intermittent fasting comes along with a wide range of benefits that can be achieved by having food items low or without calories. Intermittent fasting is all about the time when you are eating and not how much you are eating. There is nothing fixed about the types of food that you can have while fasting. But, there are certain food items that can help you in staying full for longer periods of time, without making you feel hungry. Let's have a look at them.

Food Items

Minimally-Processed Grains

Carbs form an important part of our lives. It is not considered as the enemy when it comes to the aspect of losing weight. As you will be spending the majority of the day in fasting, it is very much important to think in a strategic way about the various ways in which you can get the required amount of calories while not making you feel excessively full. You can include whole-grain food items such as whole grain bread, crackers, and bagels. Such food items can be digested very easily and can also provide your body with easy fuel. If you are willing to work out or exercise while carrying on with your intermittent fasting routine, such food items can help you by providing the right amount of energy that you need.

Lentils

Lentils are high in fiber content. Consuming half a cup of lentils in a day can easily cover about 32% of the total requirement of fiber in a day for the body. Additionally, lentils are also a great source of iron which is very much essential for the well-being of women, especially after 50. So, if you, as a woman are willing to meet all the nutritional requirements of your body by following the routine of intermittent fasting, lentils are a must on your diet.

Seitan

If you do not want to consume protein which is derived from animal sources, you need to make sure that your diet is having a balanced amount of protein that you need. Seitan is also a great source of protein. It is often called 'wheat meat' as it is the richest protein source that can be derived from nature or plants. You can bake them and can accompany them with the kind of sauce that you love.

Hummus

Hummus is often considered as the tastiest and the creamiest dips that are available for mankind. It is another great source of protein that is plant-based. It can effectively boost up the nutritional content of various types of staples such as sandwiches – just apply some hummus along with veggies and enjoy. If you want you can also make your very own hummus, just remember that the secret key to the perfect hummus is tahini and garlic.

Berries

If you starting with intermittent fasting, you need to ensure that you are having smoothies that are made from berries. For instance, you can use strawberries which are a great source of Vitamin C. having one full cup of strawberries is enough for fulfilling your overall requirement of Vitamin C. You can also easily deal with all your cravings by preparing some homemade smoothies by using berries along with other fruits. The best thing about smoothies is that when you consume them you are actually having the goodness of several food items all at one time. Thus, you can easily improve your total nutrition intake.

Potatoes

Similar to whole bread, potatoes are really good for your health. They can provide you with quick energy as they can be digested very easily without any kind of extra effort. But, while consuming potatoes, make sure that you do not have them all alone. Try to pair them up with some kind of food item, which is a great source of protein. You can also have potatoes as your snack right after getting done with your workout. Additionally, your gut consists of some bacteria of good nature that readily help in keeping up with a healthy system of digestion. Potatoes can help in maintaining the health of the good bacteria as well.

Fortified Milk

The ideal and recommended calcium intake for adults is around 1000 mg. every day. This can be achieved by consuming about three glasses of milk every day. With a really reduced window of feeding, the opportunities of drinking this much milk might turn out to be scarce. So, it is of utter importance to lay stress on food items that are rich in calcium. Vitamin D fortified milk can help in enhancing the capability of the body to absorb calcium and also helps in keeping the bones strong. For boosting up your daily intake of calcium, you can combine milk with smoothies or breakfast cereal. You can also have them all alone along with your daily meals. If you do not like having milk, you can look out for non-dairy calcium sources such as tofu.

Papaya
During the last final hours of your fasting period, you are most likely to start feeling hungry, specifically when you start with the process as a beginner. This feeling of hunger might result in overeating in huge quantities during the phase of eating. As you overeat, you might end up feeling lethargic and bloated. Papaya comes along with a unique enzyme known as papain. This enzyme acts upon the proteins and helps them in breaking down easily. You can include papaya in your protein-rich meals that will help in easing the process of digestion. It can also help in making bloat manageable in nature.

Nuts
Make up some room in your kitchen cabinet for some mixed types of nuts as nuts can readily help in getting rid of any kind of body fat. It also helps in improving the length of your life. Nuts have also been found to help in reducing the various risks that are linked with type 2 diabetes, cardiovascular diseases, along with mortality.

Fish
According to the recent Dietary Guidelines, you need to include a minimum of 8 ounces of fish in your per week diet and this is obviously for a positive reason. Fish are great sources of healthy fats and protein. It also comes along with the adequate amount of Vitamin D.

As you start fasting, fish tends to become even more essential for your diet because with only a single type of dish, you can provide your body with a complete bucket of essential nutrients. Moreover, fish also helps in enhancing the health of your brain.

Avocado

Many of you might feel skeptical after finding avocado in this list but it is actually a very healthy food item, regardless of it being high in calories. Avocado contains monosaturated nature of fat which comes with the power of making you feel full. It also imparts great satiety levels. It has been found from various studies that if you are willing to stay full for more time, adding some slices of avocado to your meal can easily help you out. This option is really a handy one for all those who want to fast for hours. It can easily help you in effectively dealing with all your cravings at the time of fasting and will prohibit you from consuming any kind of unhealthy snacks.

Cruciferous Vegetables

Vegetables such as broccoli, cauliflower, and Brussels sprouts are a great source of fiber. As you start with your routine of intermittent fasting, it is of utmost importance to include an adequate amount of fiber in your daily diet. This can help you in dealing with the problems of constipation. It can also provide you with the surety of regular bowels. Fiber also helps in inducing satiety and thus, can make you feel full for a long time. If you are deciding to fast for the next twelve hours or sixteen hours, feeling full is a must for getting the ultimate results of intermittent fasting.

Drinks

Beverages might turn out to be the life-saver whenever it comes to a situation of fighting with your hunger pangs along with cravings at the time of fasting. You can consume certain drinks that can help in enhancing the overall benefits of intermittent fasting. Let's have a look at them.

Water

You can and also should drink water during your periods of fasting. Water is always taken to be a great choice for an entire day, every day. You can have sparkling water or still water according to your choice. If you are getting bored of drinking normal water, you can add a few drops of lemon juice to your water. You can also try out several other variations of fun flavor such as you can infuse a pitcher of water with slices of orange or cucumber. But, you need to ensure that you are much away from any kind of sweetened water enhancer. Having artificial sweeteners with water can readily interfere with the fast.

Coffee

If you are looking out for a calorie-free beverage, black coffee is a great choice that does not have any kind of effect on the levels of insulin. You can consume normal coffee or black coffee during your fasting periods. Make sure that you do not add any milk or sweetener to it. You can add up spices like cinnamon for enhancing the overall taste. But, make sure that you monitor your experience of having coffee at the time of fasting as many people often suffer from an upset stomach or racing heart after consuming coffee at the time of fasting. Coffee can also help in keeping your blood sugar at normal levels for a long time.

Bone Broth

You can have bone broth or even vegetable broth at any time when you decide to fast for one day or more. But, do not opt for the canned broths. They come along with lots of preservatives and artificial flavoring that can have adverse effects on your fast. You can make your own broth and store it in the refrigerator and consume it when you want to.

Tea

Tea can help in naturally improving your satiety. It acts like the secret weapon which will not only make your plan of fasting much easier but will also make it successful. You can have any type of tea you want at the time of fasting such as black, green, herbal, and oolong teas. Tea helps in boosting up the effectiveness of the process of intermittent fasting by supporting probiotic balance, gut health, and also cellular health. Green tea has been specifically found out to be helpful in managing weight and improving satiety.

Apple Cider Vinegar

Apple cider vinegar comes along with various benefits and you can obviously drink it at the time of intermittent fasting. It helps in supporting healthy levels of blood sugar along with proper digestion. Moreover, recent studies have found out that apple cider vinegar can enhance the overall effects of intermittent fasting. If you do not like having apple cider vinegar alone, you can use it as a dressing for your salads during your windows of eating.

Some Common Questions

There are certain questions that always come up while talking about the drinks that can be consumed at the time of intermittent fasting.

Can I have diet soda at the time of fasting?

It is true that diet soda is free from any kind of calories but it can still inhibit the effects of intermittent fasting. They get their sweetness from various types of artificial sweeteners that can readily result in insulin response. So, it is better to avoid such drinks.

Can I have alcohol?

On the days of intermittent fasting, it is better to limit the consumption of alcohol during your windows of eating. The alcoholic beverages are rich in calories and sugar. So, having alcohol can actually break the fast. Also, alcohol affects the most when consumed in an empty stomach and this might result in some awful experiences the next day. So, try to avoid alcohol as much as possible.

CHAPTER 5

ADVICE
FOR WOMEN
OVER 50

Intermittent fasting, because of its wide range of benefits, has turned out to be a trending practice in recent years. And, when practiced in the proper way, it can provide you with some amazing results. Well, intermittent fasting can also help women who are over the age of 50, but for them, it might be a bit tough to carry on with the process just because of their age. So, for helping you in the journey, here is a list of some advice that can help you in reaching your goals of intermittent fasting easily and effectively.

Exercising Along With Fasting

Deciding to workout at the time of fasting can help you in various ways. It helps in increasing the fat burning rate. It has been found that if you even opt for some of the simplest exercises right before your breakfast instead of just exercising after having your breakfast, it can readily help in burning 25% of more body fat. When you exercise while keeping on with the fast, you can also develop more lean muscle. Having more lean muscles indicates better performance of the body. When you have more lean muscle, your body will try to burn out more calories not only at the time of exercising but throughout the entire day as your muscles will require more fuel in place of fat.

Also, as you exercise while fasting, it can readily improve the insulin sensitivity of your body. Insulin is a hormone that is responsible for looking after the glucose in your blood. But, did you know that insulin indicates your body when to start with fat accumulation? Insulin is also responsible for indicating all the muscles in the body to soak up all the glucose that is available in the blood and store it as fuel for later usage. When you keep working out at the time of your fasting window, your body will tend to become more sensitive to insulin, which means it will lead to easier weight loss, proper blood sugar levels, and also proper control over body glucose.

But, remember not to start with workout just like that at the very beginning. You will need to properly listen to the responses of your body in the first place. You are also required to get accustomed to the routine of fasting before you opt for exercising at the time of fasting. Do not overdo as you start with it as a beginner. If you think of starting with it intensely from the very beginning, it might end up in a lower blood sugar level. Notice if you are having any kind of feelings of weakness, dizziness, brain fog, etc. If you want you can also include some electrolyte drink for the beginning phase.

Keeping The Right Mindset

No matter what you do in your life, having the right mindset is of utter importance every time when you want to achieve something. Any kind of new step that you are deciding to take or a new journey that you are thinking to start, you cannot succeed in the absence of the proper mindset. Not having the proper mindset is the primary reason why most of the people fail to continue with the process of intermittent fasting. They just give up by taking the first step as they are not focused. If you are thinking about the overall process of intermittent fasting as only a single-time program, there is a 95% chance that you will fail in it. For getting the progressive nature of results from the process, you need to think about it in a different way. Set your mind in a way that makes you adopt intermittent fasting as an important process of your daily lifestyle. Be consistent with the process by making it an active part of your daily life.

Fasting After Dinner

Intermittent fasting is a very flexible process where people can decide on the type of fasting that they want to perform. You have already learned about the various types of intermittent fasting in the previous chapters. You also know the basics of all of them. Among all the various types of intermittent fasting that are available today, fasting after having your dinner is often considered as the most beneficial one. What exactly is the reason behind thinking so? The main reason behind this whole concept is obvious. As you start with the process of fasting after completing your dinner, you will have no work to do and just spend 90% of the time in your bed at night, having proper sleep. If you are following the 16/8 method of intermittent fasting, you can watch a movie or read a book for about three hours and then sleep for the remaining nine hours. You will be fasting for 12 hours continuously without having any kind of knowledge about it.

That is why the 16/8 method is often regarded as the easiest method of intermittent fasting and is also easier for all beginners. With this advice, you can bring about a change in your lifestyle and make it easier and healthier. You can also improve your adherence to the daily diet. You will also be having more control over all your cravings and hunger.

Keeping Yourself Busy

You can actually break all the barriers with this. When you get bored or have nothing to do, you will tend to look out for some snacks or some food items on which you can munch on. Boredom can very easily creep in your mind and also comes with the power of easily breaking your fast, especially with some sort of food item that is not actually healthy for you and the diet. We all love watching Netflix, isn't it? It is one of the most common scenarios when you will want to have something on which you can munch on for breaking the monotony. But, what exactly results in this form of action? The answer to this very question is nothing but dopamine. Dopamine is a hormone that can provide you with a feeling of happiness as you provide something that you want to yourself.

The feeling that you have immediately after having your favorite snacks does not only take place with you. We all experience this feeling. This hormone can readily make it tough to carry on with the fast. So, what is the solution to this? You need to keep yourself and your mind busy with something that will not be having any nature of relation to food items. Every time when you feel like having some snacks in the middle of your fast, try shifting your focus onto something like a really interesting TV show or get indulged in some serious work. The main motive is to stay as busy as you can.

Going For Satiating Meals

Right after starting with the process of fasting, you need to note that if you cannot have satiating meals, you might end up feeling demotivated no matter how hard you try to stick to your overall fasting routine. This is the only way by which 90% of the people lose their motivation for carrying on the process of intermittent fasting. As you decide all your meals that you are going to have during this period in a proper way, you can have an easy time in properly maintaining your overall fasting regime. You can think of the regular diet in this pattern:

- A very simple nature of egg recipe for your breakfast time.

- Any bland type of chicken or fish dish added with various types of veggies that will not be attracting you in any possible ways for your lunch.

- Right after getting done with your exercises, having protein supplements.

- A similar kind of bland dish for your dinner time.

In case you have enough time in your routine, you can also include various types of fruits and nuts for your snacks. This type of planning for all your meals will very obviously end up in dissatisfaction with your overall diet. You might also think of giving up the process. Additionally, this type of meal plan can also give you the worst nature of cravings. So, what can be done to it?

- You can remove breakfast from your daily meal routine. Just try to sustain on water or coffee or any other kind of drink that has low or zero calories.

- For the lunch meal, you can carry on with a similar type of band chicken of fish meal. But, this time try to pair it up with something that you really love, for instance, marinate your fish or chicken with BBQ seasoning.

- Take some sort of protein shake or supplement after getting done with the workout session.

- If you want or if you are really willing to, you can go out for dinner. But remember that you cannot have any type of processed foods.

CHAPTER 6

COMMON MISTAKES TO AVOID

Most people face difficulty in carrying on with the process of intermittent fasting because their approach to the whole process is completely wrong. Being actively aware of the proper methods while deciding on undertaking intermittent fasting might turn out to be the main difference between failure and success. Here are some of the most common mistakes that people make while undergoing the process of intermittent fasting that needs to be avoided for getting the ultimate results.

Using The Method As A Reason For Eating Rubbish

Well, many people think of the process of intermittent fasting just like a magic pill that can solve all the problems that they are having. It is true that intermittent fasting is actually a great tool for taking complete control over your health. But it won't be able to completely cancel out your habit of having processed foods all the time. At the time of intermittent fasting, you are required to nourish the body with all types of nutrient-rich and whole food items. When your body is in the state of fasting, your body will start breaking down all the components that are damaged in nature and will use them up for providing energy. This whole process will clean up and heal your body. This also means that your body will tend to become more sensitive to the types of food that you are going to eat.

It will be great if you are having food items that are rich in nutrients and not having anything that is rubbish. Also, when you fail to nourish the body with foods that are dense in nutrients, you will go through extreme feelings of hunger as your body will be craving for nutrients. So, using this process as the key to eat rubbish is not going to help you in any way.

Restricting Calories During The Eating Phase

The primary issue that most of the people face as they start with the process of intermittent fasting is that they try to restrict their calorie intake as they break their fast. The overall point of following intermittent fasting is to properly listen to the body and continue eating until you are full. The human body is a great machine only if you permit it to do its job in the proper way. Our body releases hormones for making us feel full when it understands that it does not need any more food. When you try to restrict your calorie intake at the time of eating, you might end up eating much less than you actually need. This will ultimately result in causing various unwanted changes in your body that might not be a really good thing for you.

Trying To Do Several Things All At Once – Under Eat, Fast, and Over Train

There is a very popular saying, 'Do not try to bite off more if you cannot chew.' If you have several years by eating in a bad way and without exercising and you want to opt for intermittent fasting, it is better not to overdo things. Try to ease yourself up with the process of fasting and start training gradually. Do not just start with training five times a week, every day fasting and calorie restriction as you eat from the first day. This overall combination might result in various types of serious problems. Your body needs a little amount of physical stress but stressing too much might result in chronic issues.

Getting Obsessed With Eating Windows And Timings

One of the primary benefits of intermittent fasting is that it can teach you to understand your body. You will learn to understand what is meant by real hunger of the body which is something that generally occurs after every 18-24 hours and not after every 3-4 hours. Your body will be dictating when you need to eat and not the ticking clock. If you try to focus only on the time periods, you will only end up counting down the total hours until which you can consume food. You are never going to learn how to understand the signals of your body.

Not Having Enough Water

When your body enters the state of fasting, it begins to break down all the damaged components and thus detoxifies your body. It is of utter importance that you throw all of these toxins out of your body by drinking enough water. As you start fasting, try to have as much water as you can have. Also, drinking water throughout your period of fasting can help in making you feel full which is really important as you start with intermittent fasting.

Allowing Fasting To Rule Over Your Life

We all love the company of our family and friends. But, as you start with the process of intermittent fasting, you might get inclined to cancel dinner with friends or any party only because you are fasting. In this way, it might turn out to be not so enjoyable for the long term. Do not allow the fasting periods to rule over your life. Try shifting your routine backward or forward only by a few hours on those days when you have got some sort of plans with your family or friends. Intermittent fasting is much more than a program; it is a lifestyle that needs to be properly mingled with your regular life. It is flexible in nature and so there is no meaning of canceling all your social plans. Just alter your routine a bit and you are good to go.

Overeating During The Eating Phase

It is very easy to overeat right after you are done with your fasting period as you might feel hungry or just want to justify yourself that you are actually filling up the calories that have been lost. This whole thinking might backfire if you are practicing intermittent fasting for losing weight. So, try to prepare some healthy meals as your fast ends and try to keep as many whole food items as possible in the diet. Do not overeat than you usually do and try keeping it normal.

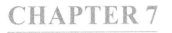

CHAPTER 7

EXERCISES TO
LOSE WEIGHT

Carrying around excessive weight always feels uncomfortable and moreover it can impact your overall health. The rates of obesity have reached new heights in the past few years. Obesity can be regarded as the storehouse of all types of diseases and thus can lead to numerous chronic health-related problems. The most common problems that arise from obesity are diabetes, heart diseases, several types of cancer, stroke, and others. A person can lose excess body weight by limiting the total calorie intake via their diet. The second way of dealing with it is by burning down extra calories with the help of exercise.

Benefits Of Exercise

The most effective way of losing weight is by combining your regular healthy diet with exercise in place of just focusing on calorie restriction. Exercise comes with the power of preventing and even reversing the effects of various diseases. As you start with exercising, you can easily lower the level of cholesterol along with blood pressure of your body which can help in preventing the chances of a heart attack. Exercise can also prevent the development of various types of cancers like breast cancer and colon cancer. It can also provide you with a sense of well-being along with confidence. Thus, it can lower the rates of depression and anxiety.

Exercise is also very helpful for losing weight and also for maintaining the loss of weight. It can help in improving your body's metabolism. With daily exercising, you can also increase and maintain your lead muscle mass which directly helps in increasing the total number of calories that you can burn in a day.

How Much Exercise Is Required For Losing Weight?

For reaping all the health-related benefits of exercising, it is always suggested that you engage yourself in some sort of aerobic exercise for a minimum session of 20 minutes for at least 3 times every week. But, if possible by you, you can easily extend the session more than 20 minutes that will actually help you in losing weight. When you include only 10-15 minutes of very moderate exercise, for example, walking or jogging for a mile, on a regular basis, it can help you in burning almost 100 extra calories. As you burn around 700 calories every week, it can equate to almost 10 lbs. of weight loss all throughout the course of the year.

Including Exercise Into Your Daily Routine

The amount of exercise that you can actually incorporate in your daily life values more than you perform it in one session. That is the reason why bringing about small changes in your regular routine can bring about a big difference in the size of your waistline. You can consider several healthy habits that you can include in your lifestyle such as:

- Riding your cycle or walking to your workplace.

- Omitting the elevator and taking the stairs.

- Parking your car at far away distances and walk along the distance in between.

Is It Possible To Exercise While Fasting?

If you are practicing intermittent fasting for losing weight or for any other reasons and you are willing to get along with your workout routine, there are certain pros and cons that you need to consider. Some research depicted that if you exercise at the time of fasting, it can affect the biochemistry of your muscles. It might also affect the body's metabolism that is directly linked to a steady level of blood sugar and sensitivity to insulin.

Some research suggests that exercising while fasting helps in depleting the stored form of carbohydrates, also known as glycogen, and thus you will be burning more amount of stored fat. Also, exercising with an empty stomach helps in speeding up the fat-burning process. So, it can be said that exercising while fasting comes with mixed type of support, where some say that it is good for health while some say it is not.

Thinking About The Timing

For making your workout session more effective in nature at the time of fasting, you are required to think about the time which is ideal for you. You need to find out whether you should opt for working out during, before, or right after the window of eating. Working out right before the eating window is ideal for those people who perform their best at the time of working out on an empty stomach. People who cannot perform their exercise with an empty stomach can opt for exercising during the eating window. Such people can effectively capitalize on the nutrition of post-workout. And, if you think you can get the best out of yourself right after fueling, you can opt for exercising after having your meal. No matter the time that you choose, try to decide it only after listening to the responses of the body. You can experiment with the various time slots and find out when your body performs the best.

How To Carry On With Safe Exercising At The Time Of Fasting

The success rate of any program of exercise or weight loss depends completely on the extent of how safe it is for sustaining over the long run. If your aim is to reduce your body fat percentage and also maintain your level of fitness while performing intermittent fasting, you are required to be in the safe zone. Let's have a look at some of the tips.

Having a meal close to your workout session: The timing of your meal can play a very big role in your workout session. The key to reaping all the benefits of a workout session is to time your meal close to the workout session. This way your body can easily tap in the stored glycogen in the body for fueling your session of workout. Also, you can include some protein supplements right after working out for gaining more lean muscles.

- **Staying hydrated:** Fasting does not mean that you cannot have water. Drinking more water while exercising at the time of fasting is always recommended.

- **Keeping up the electrolytes:** It is very important to keep up your electrolytes at the time of working out. You can try out coconut water for replenishing the electrolytes. Moreover, it is very low in calorie count and also tastes good. Opting for energy drinks such as Gatorade is not recommended as they come with high sugar content. So, it is better to avoid them as much as possible.

- **Keeping the duration and intensity low:** If you try to push your body too hard from the very beginning, it might result in dizziness and fatigue. If you cannot take up the load, just take a break. There is no need to be forceful on your body. You need to properly listen to your body if you want to yield the best results. Try to reduce the duration of your workout session during the first few weeks.

- **Considering the fast type:** The type of fast that you are performing has a lot to do with your workout session. For instance, if you are practicing an intermittent fast for 24 hours, you need to keep the intensity of your exercise as low as possible. If you are doing 16/8 fast, you can opt for the hardcore exercises as you can rest your body during the 16 hours window.

Various Types Of Exercises

The type of workout that you pick up for losing weight has a lot to do with the end results. Also, you need to choose something that you really enjoy so that you can stick to it as your daily routine.

- **Aerobics:** Despite the type of workout program that you implement in your routine, it is of utter importance that you include some sort of cardiovascular or aerobic exercise in your routine. It can help in getting the rate of your heart up and can also pump up your blood. You can start with jogging, walking, cycling, dancing, or swimming. You can also opt for any kind of fitness machines such as a stair stepper, treadmill, and others.

- **Weight training:** The biggest advantage that comes along with weight training is that, besides losing fast, you can also build up your muscles. When you have more muscles, you can burn calories much more easily. You need to work on all the major groups of muscles 3 times a week. The major muscle groups include back, abs, calves, chest, biceps, triceps, traps, shoulders, forearms, hamstrings, and quads.

Before Starting With Your Exercise Program

If you are thinking about exercising while fasting, it is always recommended to talk to your doctor at first. If you are having certain conditions such as diabetes, lung disease, heart disease, arthritis, and kidney disease, make sure that you go through a proper checkup right before starting with the program. As you start with the program, try to notice the signals that your body is giving out. Try to push yourself a bit every day to improve your level of fitness. Do not just jump into some sort of hardcore exercise from the first day.

CHAPTER 8

HOW TO MANAGE MENOPAUSE

The phase of menopause starts from the age of the late 40s or from the early 50s for the majority of women. Menopause generally lasts for some years. But, the time period of menopause is not at all smooth. It has been found that almost 63% of women go through the symptoms that are related to menopause. The symptoms of menopause are varying in nature. Let's have a look at some of the most common symptoms of menopause.

- **Irregular periods:** The early onset of menopause can be identified by periods at irregular intervals.

- **Dryness:** Women might suffer from vaginal dryness.

- **Night sweats:** Sudden sweating at nighttime.

- **Mood swings:** This is a very common symptom that includes changing of mood from good to bad and again from bad to good.

- **Gain in body weight:** There might be a sudden increase in overall body weight.

Symptoms, such as changes in the cycle of menstruation vary from women to women. Generally, you will be experiencing some irregular nature of periods right before they tend to end. The skipping of periods at the time of menopause is very common. The cycle of menstruation might skip one month and then return again, or might skip several months and then begin with normal monthly cycles after a few months. The cycle of periods will also tend to be shorter than usual. Also, women who are going through menopause have higher chances of developing various diseases such as diabetes, heart disease, obesity along with osteoporosis.

Eating Food Items Rich In Vitamin D And Calcium

During menopause, hormonal changes take place. This might result in the weakening of the bones. Thus, it can also increase the risk of developing osteoporosis. Vitamin D and calcium are often linked with good health of bones. So, you are required to include enough of all these nutrients within your daily diet. Proper intake of Vitamin D in women who are going through menopause is also linked with a lesser risk of any kind of hip fractures because of the weak nature of the bones. You can find various food items that are rich in calcium content such as milk, cheese, and yogurt. Fresh green vegetables such as spinach, kale, and collard greens come with high quantities of calcium. You can get the same from beans, sardines, beans, and various other food items. You can also opt for calcium-fortified food items such as fruit juice, alternatives of milk, and certain types of cereals.

Sunlight is regarded as the primary source of Vitamin D as it can be produced by our skin when it gets exposed to sunlight. But, with growing age, the capability of the skin for producing Vitamin D from sunlight tends to decrease. In case you do not like being in the sunlight for a long time, you can opt for Vitamin D supplements and various food items that are rich in Vitamin D content. You can have oily fish, cod liver oil, eggs, and Vitamin D fortified food items. So, for dealing with weak bones at the time of menopause, having a proper amount of Vitamin D and calcium in your diet is very important.

Maintaining And Achieving Healthy Body Weight

A very common symptom at the time of menopause is weight gain. This generally results from changes in hormones, lifestyle, genetics, and aging. When you an gain excessive amount of body fat, specifically around your waist, it increases the risk of developing various diseases like diabetes and heart disease. The symptoms of menopause might also get affected because of excessive body weight. It has been found that women who are able to shed almost 10% - 15% of their body weight at the time of menopause can easily eliminate the chances of having night sweat and hot flashes. So, it is very important to maintain your body weight for dealing with the various symptoms of menopause.

Consuming Lots Of Veggies And Fruits

When you have a diet that is rich in veggies and fruits, you can easily prevent various symptoms of menopause. Vegetables and fruits come with low-calorie count and can help you in feeling full easily. So, it can be said that vegetables and fruits are great for losing weight and maintenance of the same. Fruits and vegetables can also help in dealing with various types of heart diseases. Having fruits and vegetables daily is important especially after menopause as the risk of developing heart disease also tends to increase. This is probably because of the various factors like gain in weight, age, or reduced levels of estrogen. Also, having fruits and veggies can help in dealing with the loss of bones.

Avoiding Trigger Foods

There are certain types of food items that can effectively trigger the symptoms of menopause such as night sweats, mood swings, and hot flashes. They are most likely to trigger the symptoms when consumed at night. Some of the most common triggers include alcohol, spicy and sugary food items, and caffeine. You can try to keep a diary of symptoms. If you think that some particular food item is triggering your symptoms of menopause, you can reduce the consumption of such food items or completely avoid them.

Exercising Regularly

Although there is not an adequate amount of evidence for supporting that exercising can help in dealing with night sweats and hot flashes. But, it can help in dealing with other problems. It helps in improving your metabolism and energy, results in healthier bones and joints, better nature of sleep, and reduced stress. One study found out that regular exercising for about 3 hours every week for one complete year can help in improving the mental and physical health along with the overall life quality of menopausal women. It can also help in preventing various diseases such as heart disease, cancer, type 2 diabetes, high blood pressure, stroke, osteoporosis, and obesity.

Eating Food Items Rich In Phytoestrogens

Phytoestrogens are the plant compounds that occur naturally and can mimic the overall effects of estrogen in our bodies. Thus, they can help in balancing all the hormones. High intake of this compound in the Asian countries like Japan is regarded as the primary reason why women going through menopause in such places experience hot flashes rarely. There are various foods that are rich in phytoestrogens such as tofu, soybeans, tempeh, linseeds, flaxseeds, beans, and sesame seeds. But, the overall content of phytoestrogens in the food items depends on the methods of processing. It has been that diets that are high in soy can help in reducing the levels of cholesterol, blood pressure, reduced severity of the symptoms of menopause such as night sweats and hot flashes among all those women who are undergoing menopause.

Drinking Enough Water

Women are very likely to experience dryness at the time of menopause. This is mainly because of the decrease in the levels of estrogen. For dealing with such symptoms, you can drink around 10-12 glasses of water every day. It also helps in reducing the feeling of bloating that can result because of the hormonal changes. Additionally, water helps in dealing with weight gain and also aids in the loss of weight by making you feel full. Water can also increase the metabolism of your body. Drinking around 500ml of water about half an hour before having your meal can help you in consuming 14% fewer calories while having the meal.

Reducing Processed Foods And Refined Sugar

When you have a diet plan which is high in sugar and refined carbs, it can result in sharp dips and rises in the level of blood sugar and thus making you feel irritable and tired. In fact, it has been found that meals that are very high in refined carbs content can readily increase the overall risk of developing depression in women who just finished off with their menopause. Also, diets that are full of processed foods can affect the health of your bones. So, for better health of the bones, it is necessary to keep out processed foods and refined sugar from your daily diet.

Not Skipping Meals

It is very important to have regular meals as you are going through the period of menopause. When you indulge in irregular eating patterns, it can worsen certain symptoms of menopause and can also hinder all the efforts of weight loss. It is essential to keep all your nutritional requirements on point while going through menopause.

Eating Foods Rich In Protein

Regularly having protein-rich foods can help in the prevention of losing all the lean muscle that generally results because of aging. It has been found from a study that consuming protein all throughout the day can slow down the loss of muscles that result from aging. Also, besides maintaining lean muscle mass, protein-rich foods also help in losing weight as they help on making you feel full and also increase the total calories which are burnt. You can get enough protein from food items such as fish, meat, eggs, dairy, nuts, and legumes.

Dealing With Night Sweats

You can opt for various strategies for dealing with night sweats.

Try to dress in light clothes at night.
Opt for layered bedding so that it gets easier for you to

remove them at night.

Sleep by keeping an electric fan beside you.

Try to drink cool water all throughout the course of the night at regular intervals.

You can keep an ice pack right under your pillow so that you can turn over the pillow at times for making sure that your head is resting on the cool surface all the time.

Practicing Techniques Of Relaxation

You can start with techniques of relaxation such as paced breathing, deep breathing, massage, progressive relaxation of muscles, and guided imagery for helping yourself with the various symptoms of menopause. You need to stay relaxed for controlling night sweats and hot flashes.

Quit Smoking

Smoking can readily increase the risks of developing stroke, heart disease, cancer, osteoporosis, and several other health-related problems. Moreover, it can readily increase the severity of hot flashes and night sweats. Also, smoking can bring in the early onset of menopause.

Dealing With Urinary Problems

Many women develop urinary and bladder problems at the time of menopause. This is mainly because of the lower levels of estrogen that results in weakening of the urethra. Some women might even find it very difficult to hold their urine for a long time without going to the bathroom. This is known as urinary urge incontinence. There are also high chances of urine leaking when you cough, laugh or sneeze. This is known as urinary stress incontinence. For dealing with all these, you need to reduce or avoid having caffeine, taking medication, physical therapy, or even surgery, depending on the condition. You can also consult your doctor if the condition worsens.

Reducing Anxiety And Depression

At the time of menopause, the chances of developing anxiety and depression increase. This is mainly caused because of hormonal changes. You might go through feelings of sadness as changes occur in your body. Also, anxiety and depression can worsen the symptoms of menopause. You need to limit the consumption of alcohol as it can readily result in depression. Also, getting enough sleep can help.

Dealing With Mood Swings

A very common symptom of menopause is mood swings. Women might feel irritated or disturbed with even the smallest things. You need to keep yourself active to help deal with mood swings. If you are not active enough, try finding out ways in which you can be active. Also, do not try to take excessive duties at once. Look out for the positive ways in which you can ease your symptoms of stress.

When To See A Doctor

If the symptoms of menopause are bothering you, try consulting with your doctor. While talking about your problems make sure to discuss all the symptoms that you are facing and also the extent of the same. Also, talk with the doctor if you have undergone any kind of treatment for dealing with the symptoms of menopause before.

CHAPTER 9

HOW INTERMITTENT FASTING SLOWS DOWN AGING

No one can deny the fact that glowing and youthful skin can help in making you look more beautiful. No matter what kind of cosmetics or how expensive treatments you opt for, nothing can provide you with a similar result of having a naturally healthy glowing skin. In actuality, a sane kind of mind and a healthy body is all that we need to look beautiful. But, most of us end up ignoring the condition of our health. Our inner health gets reflected on our faces. In simple terms, you tend to be what you eat and the skin is the mirror of your health. It can reflect anything that you feed it with. The foundation of youthful and healthy skin is our metabolism.

What Causes Aging?

Is there are any kind of path available for slowing down aging without the need to go under the incision knife or without buying expensive face creams that are way too expensive? Well, the answer to this question is yes! But, the first step is to know why the process of aging takes place. Presently, the most accepted theory regarding aging is the theory of free radicals. The free radicals are unstable, oxygen-rich molecules that get produced by the process of oxidation. The process takes place naturally as our body works. The free radicals get neutralized naturally by the antioxidants. The antioxidants also fight off the pathogens.

But, at times, there are excessive numbers of free radicals in our bodies. This generally happens as our body gets exposed to environmental pollutants, cigarette smoke, ozone, radiation, inflammation, stress, and constipation. The natural levels of antioxidants in the body are unable to keep up with the free radicals. As the free radicals are of highly reactive nature, they start with the process of bonding with the body cells and thus resulting in damage. They are effective in breaking apart all the healthy form of tissues and results in blocked arteries, impaired memory, and wrinkles, the most common signs of aging. While our body produces various enzymes for guarding against the damage of free radicals, antioxidants also provide a great defense system for the body.

Mitochondria And Aging

We all have heard about mitochondria in our school which is most commonly known as the powerhouse of the cell. They are the structures responsible for producing energy in the cells that can also change their structure in regard to the demand for energy. It has been found that the capacity of the mitochondria seems to reduce with age. This ultimately affects the total amount of energy that is consumed by our body which brings in the signs of aging in the cells. That is why human beings tend to feel lethargic and tired with growing age. But, there are certain triggers that can help in maintaining the youthful state of the mitochondria. Intermittent fasting is one such trigger.

Intermittent Fasting As The Youth Fountain

It has been found that restriction of calories helps in improving longevity as it can keep mitochondria in its youthful condition. During the youthful state of the mitochondria, they can have a better form of communication with the other cellular parts which are actually critical in nature for maintaining various bodily functions. If mitochondria can be locked up in a single state, the effects of intermittent fasting can be blocked only on longevity. Intermittent fasting improves longevity by this very phenomenon of mitochondria. No one knows exactly the reason why this whole thing happens, but, science is not of conclusive nature.

Intermittent fasting is often regarded as the most effective way of restricting calorie intake. During the youthful state of the cell mitochondria, organisms have the tendency to live longer. So, it can be said that intermittent fasting also comes with benefits far beyond weight loss alone. Also, intermittent fasting helps in dealing with inflammation and also helps in reducing oxidative stress.

Does Fasting Really Help?
Intermittent fasting is a form of healthy fasting that helps our body to maintain a proper and healthy balance. Intermittent fasting for losing weight can readily affect our overall health. The signs of it are easily visible on the skin as you keep on practicing. It has been found that intermittent fasting improves the metabolism of our body which ultimately results in healthy skin and a healthy body. Thus, it is evident that intermittent fasting can help in improving our lifespan. Calorie restriction helps in boosting the overall immunity of the body as well.

How Does It Affect Skin Health?
At the time of fasting, our body tends to starve for a long period of time and this ultimately results in various metabolic changes. Our body gets the required amount of energy from the consumed food. While

there is an absence of food, the body relies on the stored body fats for deriving energy and this whole process is called gluconeogenesis. Our body tends to extract the required glucose from various non-carbohydrate sources like amino acids. Also, while fasting, there is a rise in the levels of pyrimidine and purines which helps in increasing the antioxidant level. This, in turn, helps in improving the health of your skin along with the overall health of the body. Also, when the level of antioxidants increases, it helps in maintaining a proper balance at the time of starving. This is often regarded as the natural mechanism of the body for dealing with the problems of starvation. It also helps in filling up the loss that was caused because of the free radicals and oxidative stress.

Intermittent Fasting And Inflammation

There are various ways by which intermittent fasting helps in slowing down the process of aging. The very first way by which intermittent fasting deals with aging is by reducing inflammation in the body. Intermittent fasting helps in reducing brain inflammation and it also imparts a similar kind of effect on other tissues of the body. Inflammation is a defense mechanism of the body that naturally occurs when any kind of threat is detected by the body's immune system, such as toxic compound, pathogen, or damaged molecule. But, when inflammation tends to appear more than usual or tends to get out of hands, it can result in chronic nature of inflammation and thus resulting in various types of diseases and tissue damage. Too much inflammation in the body can result in atherosclerosis, cardiovascular diseases, rheumatoid arthritis, type 2 diabetes, and also some types of cancer. Thus, intermittent fasting helps in checking the level of inflammation in the body and results in a healthy body for a long time.

Intermittent Fasting And Ketones

In the state of fasting, our body is deprived of the required amount of glucose which generally comes after consumption of protein and carbohydrates. The most preferred source of the body for energy is glucose but while fasting, our body is forced to utilize some alternative fuel source. When there is an absence of glucose in the body, our body breaks down the stored fat in the liver and turns it into a ready source of energy which is known as ketones. Ketones are sent to the mitochondria and are used up by the heart, muscles, and brain.

There are certain parts of our body, specifically in the brain, that are unable to utilize the ketones and look out for glucose for their functioning. This very glucose gets supplied by the process of protein breakdown along with the breakdown of fat glycerol by the process of gluconeogenesis which has already been discussed in the previous sections. Ketones come along with certain benefits of anti-aging and let's discuss it by taking Alzheimer's disease as an example. Alzheimer's disease is a disease that is linked to the metabolism of glucose. This is the very reason why Alzheimer's is often known as type 3 diabetes. With the help of bypassing the overall shortcomings of much less than the optimal metabolism of glucose, ketones are capable of directly supplying the brain with all the energy that it needs and also helps in improving the cognitive nature of functions of all those who are suffering from Alzheimer's disease.

It has been found from a study that the process of ketosis resulted in enhanced memory in all those people who are going through the early onset of Alzheimer's disease or MCI (mild cognitive impairment). Also, ketosis which is induced through the changes in diet can help in improving the memory of elderly people who has cognitive impairment. Thus, it can be said that intermittent fasting which helps in inducing the process of ketosis can help in mitigating the effects of brain aging.

Hormesis

Evidence has depicted that practicing intermittent fasting daily can help the cells in becoming more volatile against cellular stress. This very cellular volatility is a result of hormesis which is the process of describing various natures of biological responses to cellular stress. Two common examples of hormesis are consuming vegetables and exercising. Both working out and certain phytochemicals that are present in vegetables can result in a certain degree of stress for the body. But, vegetables and exercise are both essential in nature as the response of the body to this form of stress is positive in nature. Intermittent fasting can also be regarded as an example of hormesis. Excessive fasting will result in catabolism of the muscle tissues and ultimately result in death.

When a little amount of stress is given to the body on a regular basis, it can easily avoid all the related negative effects and might end up in inducing the positive nature of biological responses with time. This helps in improving your volatility to oxidative nature of stress which is often regarded as one of the primary factors 0f degenerative disease and aging.

Triggers Autophagy

The term autophagy has been derived from a Greek word that indicates self-eating. It is the process of self-recycling of cellular waste. It gets increased when stress is induced in the body. With growing age, the process of autophagy tends to slow down and thus decreases the ability of the body to effectively recycle all the cells under the effect of stress. By practicing intermittent fasting, autophagy can be increased very easily which is directly linked with slowing down the aging rate as the body is kept primed for combating various natures of cellular stress. It has been found from a study that fasting for a short period of time, probably for 24 – 48 hours, can induce neural autophagy. But, does this also mean that the typical nature of intermittent fasting, probably for 16 – 23 hours, can also induce the process of autophagy?

To date, all the researches regarding autophagy and fasting have primarily focused on fasts for 24 – 48 hours. This is completely based in regard to that autophagy increases side by side along with ketosis which generally takes around 24 – 48 hours for getting induced. But, ketosis can also occur much before the fasting period of 24 hours and sometimes without even fasting. Thus, it can be said that intermittent fasting can induce ketosis and thus resulting in autophagy.

Bottom Line

Intermittent fasting can help you in many more ways than you can actually think. It not only permits the body to burn down the excess stored fat but also helps in keeping you healthier. It also slows down the process of aging. Additionally, it can also deal with inflammation in the body and thus helps in improving your age. By eating within a specified window of time on a regular basis, you can activate a wide range of anti-aging mechanisms in your body. So, what are you waiting for? Start with intermittent fasting today and make your skin glow brighter and make your body younger with growing age.

CHAPTER 10

EASY RECIPES FOR INTERMITTENT FASTING

For making everything much easier for you, here are some recipes that you can follow while practicing intermittent fasting. Intermittent fasting recipes are nothing fancy and are more or less like the normal diet that you follow daily.

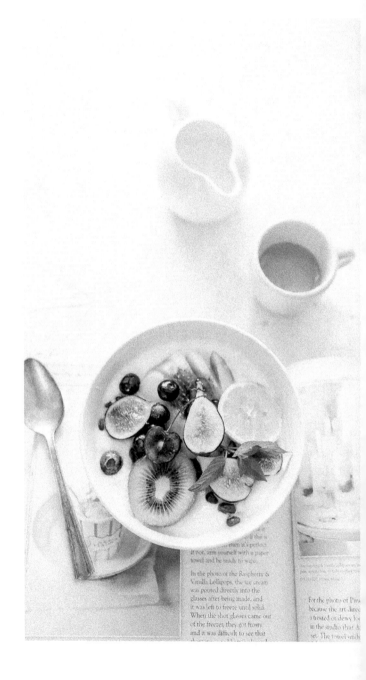

it not, arm yourself with a paper
towel and be ready to wipe.

In the photo of the *Raspberry &
Vanilla Lollipops*, the ice cream
was pooled directly into the
glasses after being made, and
it was left to freeze until solid.
When the shot glasses came out
of the freezer, they got frosty
and it was difficult to see that

For the photo of *Piru*
because the art direc
a frosted or dewy lo
in the studio that d
set. The towel unfo

Breakfast

Breakfast is a very important meal in intermittent fasting as it might be the first meal of yours after fasting for a long period of time. So, let's have a look at some easy recipes for breakfast.

Breakfast Burrito

Total Prep & Cooking Time: 30 minutes
Yield: 2 servings
Nutritional facts: Calories: 410 | Protein: 14g | Fat: 37g
| Carbs: 8g | Fiber: 4g

Ingredients:

- Two large eggs
- Four strips of bacon (cooked)
- One sliced tomato
- Half cup of avocado (sliced)
- Two tbsps. of each
    - Heavy cream
    - Mayonnaise
- One cup chopped lettuce
- Two tsps. butter
- Salt & pepper

Method:

1. Break the eggs in a mixing bowl and whisk well. Add heavy cream to the whisked eggs. Add pepper & salt for seasoning.
2. Take a skillet and heat it on medium flame. Add one tsp. of butter to the skillet.
3. Add half of the whisked egg mixture to the skillet and tilt the skillet either side by side or back and forth for making sure that the entire base of the skillet gets covered by the egg mixture.
4. Cover the skillet by using a lid and allow the egg to cook for one minute or so.
5. Try to shake the skillet back and forth and flip the crepe with utmost care by using a flat spatula.
6. After the egg gets cooked perfectly, place it on a

paper napkin or towel for getting rid of excess oil.

7. For the remaining egg mixture, repeat the same steps.

8. Apply some mayonnaise to the crepe and add tomatoes, lettuce, bacon, and avocado.

9. Add pepper & salt for seasoning.

10. Carefully roll the crepes. Serve hot.

Note: For ensuring that the crepes do not stick to the base of the skillet, use a non-stick skillet.

Parmesan Spinach Baked Eggs

Total Prep & Cooking Time: 50 minutes
Yield: 4 servings
Nutritional facts: Calories: 130 | Protein: 12g | Fat: 11g | Carbs: 5g | Fiber: 2g

Ingredients:
- Two tsps. extra virgin olive oil
- Half cup grated parmesan cheese
- One small tomato (diced)
- Four cups of spinach
- Two cloves of garlic (minced)
- Four large eggs
- Salt & pepper

Method:
1. Set your oven temperature to 360 degrees Fahrenheit and preheat.
2. Take a casserole baking tray and coat it with cooking spray.
3. Take a large pan and heat it on high flame. Add olive oil to the pan.
4. Start adding spinach and garlic to the pan once the oil heats up. Properly cook the spinach until it wilts completely. Drain out the excess liquid after removing the pan from heat.
5. Add parmesan cheese to the cooked spinach and mix well.
6. Layer the spinach and cheese mixture on the casserole tray evenly by using a spoon.
7. Make small pits on the layered spinach for making space for the eggs.
8. Bake the spinach and egg for about 20 mins. or until the eggs cook properly.
9. Serve with tomatoes on the top.

Smoothie Protein Bowl

Total Prep & Cooking Time: 10 minutes
Yield: 2 servings
Nutritional facts: Calories: 280 | Protein: 11g | Fat: 19g
| Carbs: 40g | Fiber: 3g

Ingredients:

- One ripe frozen banana
- One tbsp. of each
   –Almond butter or cashew butter
   –Honey
- Two tbsps. of flax seeds or hemp
- Half cup of Greek yogurt
- One tsp. vanilla
- One scoop protein powder
- One cup of coconut water

For toppings:

- Slices of banana
- Raspberries
- Strawberries
- Blueberries
- Pomegranate season

Method:

1. Put together honey, ripe banana, almond butter, yogurt, flax seeds, coconut water, protein powder, and vanilla in a blender. Blend the mixture well until smooth.
2. Transfer the smoothie in serving bowls and top it with strawberries, raspberries, pomegranate, blueberries, and sliced banana.

Breakfast Muffins With Turkey Sausage

Total Prep & Cooking Time: 45 minutes
Yield: 10 servings
Nutritional facts: Calories: 152 | Protein: 14g | Fat: 10g | Carbs: 6g | Fiber: 2g

Ingredients:

- Three full cups of diced wheat bread
- Half pound turkey sausage
- Five egg whites
- Two large eggs
- Two cups cheddar cheese (shredded)
- One-fourth cup of each
    - Chopped red onion
    - Chopped green capsicum
    - Milk
- Kosher salt for seasoning

Method:

1. Set the oven temperature to 380 degrees Fahrenheit and preheat.
2. You can either use a muffin tin and coat it well with cooking spray or use paper cup liners for the muffins.
3. Take a medium-sized pan and cook well the sausage. Cook the sausage until there is no pink color in them.
4. Break down the sausages at the time of cooking by using a spatula.
5. Add chopped onion and capsicum to the ground sausage. Cook properly until soft.
6. Divide the diced bread cubes into ten muffin cups.

7. Top the bread cubes by using cooked sausage mixture. Fill the cups about three-fourth.
8. Add cheese from the top.
9. Take a mixing bowl and whisk in egg whites, egg, kosher salt, and milk. Pour the mixture over the filled muffin cups. Make sure that the ingredients in the cups get covered properly by the egg mixture.
10. Allow the muffin cups to rest for about 10 – 12 minutes. If needed, you can add in more egg mixture to the cups.
11. Bake them for about 15 – 20 minutes or until it gets set properly from the middle. Make sure that the top of the muffins gets browned.
12. Take the muffins out from the oven and allow them to rest for 5 mins. right before removing them from the cups.
13. Serve warm.

Hummus Breakfast Bowl

Total Prep & Cooking Time: 45 minutes
Yield: 2 servings
Nutritional facts: Calories: 355 | Protein: 13g | Fat: 17g
| Carbs: 35g | Fiber: 4g

Ingredients:

- One tbsp. extra virgin olive oil
- One cup kale (remove the stems and chop the leaves roughly)
- Two egg whites
- One tbsp. hummus
- One cup tomato (diced)
- Three-fourth cup of cooked quinoa or brown rice
- Two tbsps. minced bell pepper of any color
- One tsp. sunflower seeds
- Salt & pepper

Method:

1. Take a large pan and heat it over medium flame. Add olive oil to the pan.
2. Add kale to the hot oil and sauté well the kale for about 4 to 5 mins.
3. Once the kale gets cooked, add tomatoes and bell pepper to the pan. Cook the mixture for about 5 mins.
4. Take a mixing bowl and beat the eggs. Add the beaten eggs to the pan into the kale mixture.
5. Use a spatula and scramble the eggs until they are evenly cooked.
6. Take a serving bowl and place the cooked quinoa or rice in it. Add the mixture of eggs and kale over it.
7. Take a spoon of hummus and place it over the egg mixture.
8. Add sunflower seeds from the top.
9. Serve hot.

Oatmeal And Raisin Bites

Total Prep & Cooking Time: 45 minutes
Yield: 2 servings
Nutritional facts: Calories: 160 | Protein: 7g | Fat: 7g |
Carbs: 15g | Fiber: 3g

Ingredients:

- One-quarter cup of each
  - –Chopped peanuts
  - –Raisins
  - –Peanut butter
  - –Chocolate chips
- One cup of dried oats
- Half tsp. of grounded cinnamon
- Two tbsps. of honey
- One scoop vanilla flavored protein powder

Method:

1. Take a mixing bowl and mix all the ingredients together. Mix until it turns sticky.
2. Take a baking tray and place parchment paper on it. You can also use cooking spray.
3. Take a spoon of the mixture and roll it into small balls of about one-inch.
4. Place each of the balls on the baking tray with a proper gap in between.
5. Take the baking tray and place it in the refrigerator for about half an hour to ensure that the balls get firm.

Note: You can store the balls for about one week by keeping them in an air-tight container and place it in the fridge.

Egg And Ham Cups

Total Prep & Cooking Time: 35 minutes
Yield: 6 servings
Nutritional facts: Calories: 95 | Protein: 10g | Fat: 4g |
Carbs: 4g | Fiber: 1g

Ingredients:

- Three egg whites
- Three large eggs
- Twelve slices of thin ham (low sodium)
- Half cup milk
- Two chopped green onions
- Salt & pepper

Method:

1. Start by setting the temperature of the oven to 350 degrees Fahrenheit. Preheat the oven.
2. Take a muffin tray and coat it generously by using cooking spray.
3. Press each piece of ham slices and create a shape of the cup by pressing them in the muffin tin.
4. Take a mixing bowl and mix together egg whites, eggs, and milk. Whisk it properly. Add pepper and salt for seasoning.
5. Pour the egg mixture into the ham muffin cups. Make sure that the cups are not filled more than three-fourth of its size.
6. Bake the ham cups in the oven for about 20 mins. or until the eggs are properly set.
7. Cool the ham cups before serving.

Note: You can also add other vegetables to the cups for improving the flavor and nutrient content.

Avocado And Baked Eggs

Total Prep & Cooking Time: 25 minutes
Yield: 2 servings
Nutritional facts: Calories: 560 | Protein: 19g | Fat: 42g
| Carbs: 16g | Fiber: 12g

Ingredients:

- Two tbsp. fresh lime juice
- One avocado (medium-sized)
- Two large eggs
- Two tbsps. cheese (shredded)
- Salt & pepper

Method:

1. Start by setting the oven temp. to 350 degrees Fahrenheit. Preheat.
2. Take a sharp knife and cut the avocado in equal halves.
3. Scoop out some of the flesh of avocado by using a spoon for making room in the center.
4. Take a baking sheet and place the avocado halves upright.
5. Use lemon juice for brushing the avocado.
6. Crack in one egg in the center of the avocados. Add salt and pepper for seasoning.
7. Bake the avocados for about 10 mins. or until the egg cooks properly.
8. Add some cheese from the top and bake the avocados again for about 2 mins. for melting the cheese.
9. Serve hot with pepper from the top.

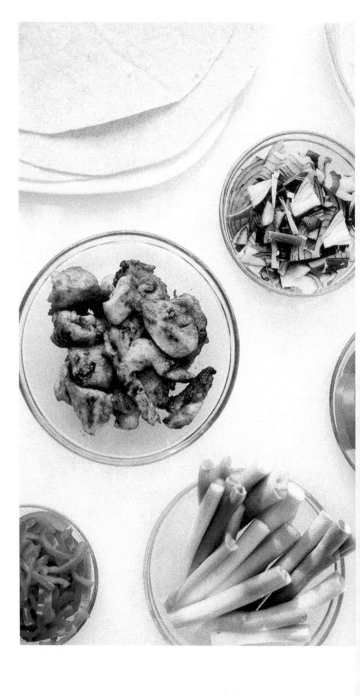

Lunch

Lunch is a very important meal in intermittent fasting. You can opt for your lunch and then continue with the fast for about 16 hours until breakfast.

Fish Tacos

Total Prep & Cooking Time: 35 minutes
Yield: 8 servings
Nutritional facts: Calories: 200 | Protein: 19g | Fat: 3g |
Carbs: 22g | Fiber: 4g

Ingredients:

For Tacos:
- One-quarter cup of each
  - Cornmeal
  - Whole wheat flour
  - Breadcrumbs
- One cup of each
  - Shredded lettuce or cabbage
  - Sour cream or Greek yogurt (non-fat)
- One diced tomato
- Two tbsps. of fresh lime juice
- Two egg whites
- Eight wheat flour tortillas or corn tortillas (about six inches in size)
- Two tbsps. taco seasoning
- Five fillets of fish (Flounder or Tilapia cut into wide strips of two inches, about four strips from each fillet)

For Taco Seasoning:
- Half tsp. of each
  - Minced dried garlic
  - Minced dried onion
- Two cups of each
  - Ground cumin seeds
  - Dried cilantro
- One tsp. of each

–Black pepper

–Oregano

–Paprika

- One tbsp. chili powder
- Salt & pepper

Method:

For Taco Seasoning:

1. Take a glass jar and mix all the ingredients for seasoning. Cover it using a lid.
2. Make sure to keep the jar away from heat, moisture, and light.

Note: Try to purchase raw herbs and spices in the dried state. Make sure that there is no f0rm of added preservatives or sodium.

For Tacos:

1. For starting with the process, set the oven temperature to 400 degrees Fahrenheit. Preheat the oven.
2. Take a baking tray and line it properly by using aluminum foil. Keep one cooking rack on top of the tray spray properly with canola oil or olive oil.
3. Take one mixing bowl and mix in breadcrumbs, cornmeal, and taco seasoning.
4. Take another bowl and add in egg whites along with lime juice. Whisk it well until it turns into a frothy mixture.
5. Use a small bowl and pour some flour in it.
6. Now, take each of the fish strips one by one and coat them in the flour for coating for sides properly.

7. Dip the flour coated fish strips in the egg white mixture. Now press the strips on the breadcrumbs mixture.
8. Place the strips on the cooking rack and bake them for 12 mins. or until they turn golden brown in color.
9. Toast the tortillas for about 30 seconds in a pan after coating it properly with cooking spray.
10. Take the tacos and place two cooked strips of fish in each.
11. Garnish the tacos with yogurt, salsa, and tomato.

Note: You can add bell peppers and cucumber for adding freshness to the tacos.

Tuna Salad

Total Prep & Cooking Time: 30 minutes

Yield: 8 servings

Nutritional facts: Calories: 75 | Protein: 14g | Fat: 1g | Carbs: 4g | Fiber: 2g

Ingredients:

- Two tbsps. lemon juice
- Five ounces of tuna cans (water-packed)
- One carrot (grated)
- One tomato (chopped)
- Half tsp. garlic powder
- Half white onion (chopped)
- Half tsp. dried dill
- One boiled egg (chopped)
- One cup Greek yogurt
- One tsp. honey
- One tsp. parsley (dried)
- One tsp. of Dijon mustard

Method:

1. Take a large mixing bowl and put in all the ingredients.
2. Mix properly and serve.

Quinoa And Ground Turkey Salad

Total Prep & Cooking Time: 20 minutes
Yield: 10 servings
Nutritional facts: Calories: 98 | Protein: 7g | Fat: 3g |
Carbs: 11g | Fiber: 3g

Ingredients:
- One and a half cup of quinoa (cooked)
- Half pound turkey sausage (ground)
- One sliced red onion
- Three sliced cucumbers (sliced into circles)
- One cup cherry tomatoes (halved)
- Two minced garlic cloves
- Half cup of each
  - Crumbles of feta cheese
  - Kalamata olives
- Two tbsps. chopped mint leaves
- One tbsp. of each
  - Fresh chopped oregano
  - Lemon juice

Method:
1. Take a large skillet and cook the sausage. Break the sausage into very small pieces while cooking.
2. Drain off excess liquid from the skillet and allow the cooked sausage to cool down properly.
3. Take a mixing bowl and mix in tomatoes, quinoa, onions, cucumber, olives, garlic, cheese crumbles, and cooked sausage. Combine well.
4. Add lemon juice to the mixture along with oregano and mint. Chill the salad before serving.

Lemon And Fish Fillets

Total Prep & Cooking Time: 35 minutes
Yield: 4 servings
Nutritional facts: Calories: 200 | Protein: 19g | Fat: 13g
| Carbs: 1g | Fiber: 4g

Ingredients:

- One tsp. of black pepper (ground)
- Three tbsps. extra virgin olive oil
- Two medium-sized lemons (one cut into wedges and one into half)
- Six ounces of flounder or cod
- Salt & pepper

Method:

1. Allow the fish to rest at room temperature for about 15 – 20 minutes.
2. Take the fish fillets and rub each side of the fillets with pepper, salt, and oil.
3. Take a large skillet and heat it over medium flame. Add olive oil to the skillet. Make sure that the oil is properly hot.
4. Add the fish fillets to the skillet and cook both sides for about 3 – 4 minutes. Cook until each side turns brown in color.
5. Now, take the halves of lemon and squeeze the juice over the fillets of fish.
6. Store the lemon juice from the skillet.
7. Take a serving plate and place the wedges on it for making a base.
8. Place the fish fillets over the lemon wedges.
9. Sprinkle leftover lemon juice from the skillet from the top.

Spring Roll Chicken Jars

Total Prep & Cooking Time: 35 minutes
Yield: 4 servings
Nutritional facts: Calories: 400 | Protein: 22g | Fat: 5g | Carbs: 75g | Fiber: 4g

Ingredients:

- One tbsp. minced ginger
- One bag coleslaw
- Two cloves of minced garlic
- One lb. ground chicken
- Half cup sweet chili sauce
- One tbsp. sesame oil
- Two tbsps. soy sauce
- Two cups cooked vermicelli noodles
- One cup thinly sliced cucumber
- One cup sliced red pepper
- One cup chopped cilantro (mint or basil can also be used)
- Sriracha and sesame seeds

Method:

1. Take a large skillet and heat it over medium flame. Add sesame oil to it.
2. Add ground chicken to the oil along with soy sauce. Cook the chicken for about four minutes.
3. Add garlic and ginger to the chicken and sauté again for 5 mins. Cook until the chicken is soft which will take about 8 mins.
4. Put the chicken in a bowl and in the same skillet, add soy sauce and coleslaw.
5. Cook until the coleslaw wilts.

6. Cook the vermicelli noodles on the side by following the packet instructions. It would roughly take around four minutes in hot boiling water.

7. Take 4 mason jars (medium-sized). Divide chili sauce in all the jars equally.

8. Place cooked chicken in the jars in equal portions followed by cooked coleslaw, red pepper, and cucumber.

9. Top the jars by using the vermicelli noodles. Add herbs, sesame seeds, and sriracha from the top before serving.

Detox Salad

Total Prep & Cooking Time: 35 minutes
Yield: 6 servings
Nutritional facts: Calories: 180 | Protein: 6g | Fat: 2g |
Carbs: 16g | Fiber: 4g

Ingredients:

- Half cup of each
    - Fresh chopped parsley
    - Almonds
- Two cups of each
    - Brussels sprouts (chopped)
    - Kale
- Florets of broccoli
- Red cabbage
- Two tbsps. sunflower seeds
- One cup chopped carrots

For dressing:

- Three tbsps. of extra virgin olive oil
- Three tsps. Dijon mustard
- Two tbsps. maple syrup or honey
- Half cup fresh lemon juice
- One tbsp. chopped ginger
- Salt & pepper

Method:

1. Take kale, florets of broccoli, red cabbage, and
   Brussels sprouts in a blending bowl and blend them
   until they are finely chopped. You might need to
   divide them into equal batches for getting them
   finely chopped.

2. Roughly chop the almonds in the food processor. Add it to the mixture of processed veggies in a mixing bowl.
3. Add sunflower seeds to the mixture and combine well.
4. Take all the ingredients for the dressing and mix them well in a mixing bowl.
5. Sprinkle the dressing generously from the top and mix well.
6. Serve cold.

Lettuce And Beef Wraps

Total Prep & Cooking Time: 30 minutes
Yield: 2 servings
Nutritional facts: Calories: 360 | Protein: 32g | Fat: 25g | Carbs: 5g | Fiber: 3g

Ingredients:
- Two tbsps. coconut oil
- One cup diced onions
- One diced red pepper
- Three lbs. ground beef
- Two tbsps. chopped cilantro
- One tsp. minced ginger
- Two tsps. cumin
- Four minced cloves of garlic
- Eight large leaves of cabbage
- Salt & pepper

Method:
1. Take a frying pan and heat it over medium flame. Add coconut oil to the pan.
2. Add onions to the pan and sauté for five minutes. Add in peppers and beef to the pan and cook properly.
3. Add pepper, salt, garlic, ginger, and cumin to the beef while cooking.
4. Take a large-sized pot and pour water in it until it is full by 3/4th. Bring the water to a boil.
5. Boil the cabbage leaves in water for about 20 secs. Allow the leaves to blanch in the hot water.
6. Take out each of the leaves and put them in ice-cold water.

7. Drain water from the leaves.
8. Place the cooked beef mixture in each of the leaves. Roll the leaves properly.

Notes: You can also use chicken or turkey in place of beef. Some extra veggies such as bell peppers and tomatoes can also be added. Serve in room temperature or light warm.

Beef Curry

Total Prep & Cooking Time: 50 minutes
Yield: 3 servings
Nutritional facts: Calories: 520 | Protein: 42g | Fat: 30g | Carbs: 16g | Fiber: 11g

Ingredients:

- One cup coconut milk
- One onion (chopped)
- One tbsp. of each
  –Ginger (grated)
  –Garlic (minced)
- One pound beef chuck (chopped)
- Two tbsps. curry powder
- One cup cilantro (chopped)
- Salt & pepper

Method:

1. Take a food processor and blend together onion, garlic, and ginger. Make a smooth paste.
2. Take a saucepan and heat it over medium flame. Add the onion paste to the pan. Cook it for about 5 mins. over low flame.
3. Add coconut milk to the saucepan and simmer it for about 10 mins.
4. Add in chopped beef to the mixture.
5. Add curry powder and salt.
6. Stir the curry well occasionally simmer it for 20 mins. Make sure the beef cooks properly.
7. Add pepper and salt according to your taste.
8. Serve hot with cilantro from the top.

Note: Canned coconut milk can also be used.

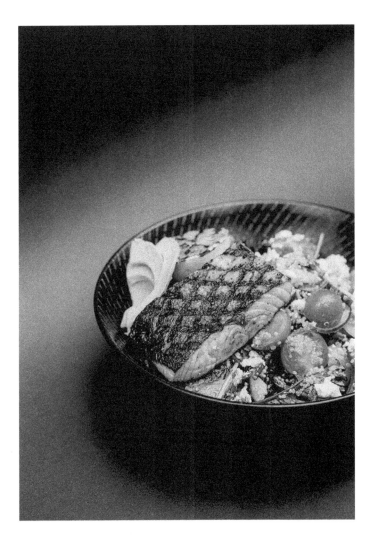

Dinner

Your dinner needs to be wholesome if you are practicing intermittent fasting. Let's have a look at some tasty dinner recipes.

Burrito Turkey Skillet

Total Prep & Cooking Time: 20 minutes
Yield: 6 servings
Nutritional facts: Calories: 360 | Protein: 32g | Fat: 16g | Carbs: 28g | Fiber: 6g

Ingredients:
- Half cup of Greek yogurt
- One pound ground turkey
- Four tortillas (whole wheat; cut into strips of one-inch size)
- One cup of each
  - Chunky salsa
  - Cheddar cheese
- One can of beans
- One tbsp. of each
  - Lime juice
  - Chili powder
- One cup of water
- One tsp. cumin (ground)
- One-fourth tsp. black pepper (ground)
- One-fourth cup cilantro (chopped)
- Salt & pepper

Method:
1. Take a large skillet and cook the turkey. Cook the turkey until it is cooked thoroughly. Try to break the turkey into pieces at the time of cooking.
2. Add salsa, beans, lime juice, and water to the cooked skillet. Season the mixture properly with pepper & salt. Add the spices – cumin and chili powder.

3. Bring the mixture to a boil and then simmer it on low flame. Thicken the sauce by simmering for about 4 – 5 mins.
4. Remove the pan from the heat. Add in the strips of tortilla.
5. Top the mixture with cheese. Cover the skillet until the cheese melts properly.
6. Add Greek yogurt along with cilantro from the top. Serve warm.

Turkey Meatloaf

Total Prep & Cooking Time: 50 minutes
Yield: 8 servings
Nutritional facts: Calories: 125 | Protein: 14g | Fat: 5g |
Carbs: 5g | Fiber: 2g

Ingredients:

- One large egg
- One pound ground turkey
- One-third cup of each
    - Ketchup
    - Chunky salsa
    - Rolled oats
- Half cup diced onions
- Salt & pepper

Method:

1. Start by setting the oven temp. to 375 degrees Fahrenheit and preheat.
2. Take a mixing bowl and add in turkey, salsa, whisked egg, and onions. Mix it well. Add pepper and salt to the turkey mixture according to your taste.
3. Take a loaf pan of 5*7 inches. Pour the turkey mixture in the loaf pan. Press the mixture evenly for setting it.
4. Bake the meatloaf for about half an hour, uncovered.
5. Take out the loaf from the pan and evenly spread out the ketchup over the loaf.
6. Bale the meatloaf again for 15 mins.
7. Allow the meatloaf to rest in the pan for about 5 mins. before taking it out.
8. You can either take out the entire load and the slice it up or you can also slice it within the pan and then place on the plates.
9. Serve warm.

Buttered Cod

Total Prep & Cooking Time: 15 minutes
Yields: 4 servings
Nutrition Facts: Calories: 280 | Protein: 28g | Carbs: 5g
| Fat: 18g| Fiber 1g

Ingredients:

For cod:

- Two lbs. of cod fillets
- Six tbsps. butter (unsalted, sliced)

For seasoning:

- One tsp. garlic powder
- One tsp. ground pepper
- Few slices of lemon
- One tsp. ground paprika
- Chopped cilantro or parsley
- Salt

Method:

1. Take a mixing bowl and mix in ground pepper, garlic powder, salt, herbs, ground paprika, and lemon slices.
2. Season the cod fillets by using the seasoning. Make sure to cover both sides of the fillets.
3. Take a large skillet and heat butter in it over medium flame.
4. Add cod fillets to the butter and cook it for about two mins.
5. Reduce the flame and turn over the fillets. Use the leftover butter over the fillets and cook again for about 5 mins.
6. Make sure that the fillets are not overcooked as it is a very mushy fish and might fall apart.
7. Serve hot with herbs and lemon juice from the top.

Broccoli And Chicken Stir-Fry

Total Prep & Cooking Time: 20 minutes
Yield: 4 servings
Nutritional facts: Calories: 260 | Protein: 32g | Fat: 19g | Carbs: 16g | Fiber: 2g

Ingredients:

- Two tsps. of each
  - Lemon juice
  - Sesame seeds
- One tbsp. of each
  - Olive oil (extra virgin)
  - Flour or cornstarch
  - Honey
- Twenty ounces fillets of chicken breast (diced)
- Three tbsps. soy sauce
- Two cups florets of broccoli
- One chopped ginger (one inch)
- Two tbsps. sesame oil
- One chopped onion
- Salt & pepper

Method:

1. Take a mixing bowl and whisk together lemon juice, soy sauce, flour, honey, and sesame oil. Mix well and keep it aside.
2. Take a large skillet or frying pan and toast the sesame seeds. While toasting, keep the flame medium-high and toast for about two mins. Keep the toasted seeds in a bowl.
3. Add some olive oil to the same skillet and heat it on medium flame. Add diced chicken to the skillet and cook until it turns golden brown in color.

4. Add in onions, pepper, broccoli, and ginger to the chicken and sauté for about 5 mins.
5. Bring down the flame to low and add the soy sauce mixture to the skillet. Toss the chicken properly so that everything gets mixed together.
6. Keep on cooking until the sauce thickens. But, make sure that you do not cook it for more than 5 mins.
7. Add toasted sesame seeds from the top before serving.

Note: You can have broccoli and chicken stir fry with quinoa or rice.

Lemon Chicken And Asparagus

Total Prep & Cooking Time: 25 minutes
Yields: 4 servings
Nutrition Facts: Calories: 230 | Protein: 28g | Carbs: 10g | Fat: 8g| Fiber 2.5g

Ingredients:

- Two sliced lemons
- One cup flour
- One pound boneless chicken breast
- Two tbsps. butter
- Two cups of chopped asparagus
- One tsp. of lemon pepper seasoning
- Chopped parsley (for topping)
- Two tbsps. honey
- Salt & pepper

Method:

1. Cover the chicken breast in a plastic wrap and pound it evenly for making the thickness to a quarter inch. Cut the pounded chicken breast into small pieces. If the chicken breast is too much in thickness, you can slice it into half.
2. Take a dish and mix together salt, pepper, and flour.
3. Toss the pieces of chicken in the flour mixture.
4. Make sure that the pieces get coated evenly.
5. Take a skillet and heat it over medium flame. Add butter to the skillet.
6. Add the chicken pieces to the skillet and sauté for about 5 mins. Sauté until the pieces turn golden brown in color.

7. Sprinkle lemon pepper seasoning on the chicken pieces as you sauté.
8. Place the chicken pieces on a plate.
9. Add asparagus to the same skillet and sauté it until crispy and the color turns to bright green. Sauté until tender.
10. Caramelize the slices of lemon by placing them in the pan over medium heat. The slices will soak up all the butter and chicken that is leftover in the pan.
11. Layer everything in a skillet by placing the cooked asparagus at the base and then followed by the cooked chicken. Add the lemon slices at the top.

Avocado Salsa And Salmon

Total Prep & Cooking Time: 20 minutes

Yields: 4 servings

Nutrition Facts: Calories: 440 | Protein: 36g | Carbs: 10g | Fat: 30g| Fiber 6g

Ingredients

For Salmon:

- Four pieces of Salmon (six ounces)
- One tbsp. oil
- Four tsps. Cajun seasoning

For Avocado Salsa:

- One diced jalapeno
- One cup diced red onion
- One tbsp. lime juice
- Two diced avocado
- One tbsp. chopped cilantro
- Salt

For Cucumber Avocado Salsa:

- Two diced avocado
- One cup diced cucumber
- One tbsp. lime juice
- One tbsp. chopped parsley
- One cup diced green onion
- Salt

Method:

1. Take a skillet and heat it over medium flame. Add oil to the skillet.

2. Season the fish with Cajun seasoning. Add the fish to the skillet and cook for about 5 – 10 mins. or until it turns golden brown in color.
3. Flip the fish and do the same.
4. For preparing the avocado salsa, mix all the ingredients together in a mixing bowl.
5. For the cucumber avocado salsa, mix together all the ingredients in a mixing bowl and toss properly.
6. Serve the fish with a salsa of your choice by the side.

Note: You can use any other fish in place of salmon such as tilapia or trout. Also, do not use both the salsa together, use any one of the two.

Grilled Chicken With Blackberry Salad

Total Prep & Cooking Time: 40 minutes
Yields: 2 servings
Nutrition Facts: Calories: 550 | Protein: 45g | Carbs: 8g
| Fat: 40g| Fiber 6g

Ingredients:

- Two large-sized breasts of chicken
- One tsp. thyme
- Two lettuce heads
- One-fourth cup of each
  - Black olives
  - Green olives
  - Olive oil
- One lemon (juiced)
- One cup fresh blackberries
- One tbsp. lemon juice
- One cup canned artichoke hearts
- Salt & pepper

Method:

1. Marinate the chicken breasts by using olive oil, thyme, salt, and lemon juice. Leave the chicken breasts to marinate for about half an hour.
2. Set your oven temp. to 400 degrees Fahrenheit and preheat.
3. Take a baking tray and place the marinated chicken breasts on it. Bake the chicken for about half an hour without any cover on top.
4. Take out the chicken and slice it into pieces of your choice.
5. Wash the lettuce heads and drain off any excess water by placing it on a paper towel.

6. Slice up the artichoke hearts after draining the liquid from it.
7. Mix the artichoke hearts with the sliced chicken in a bowl.
8. Add black olives, green olives along with the blackberries to the bowl.
9. Drizzle olive oil and lemon juice from the top.
10. Serve the salad with chicken immediately.

Sausage And Mushroom Skillet

Total Prep & Cooking Time: 35 minutes
Yields: 2 servings
Nutrition Facts: Calories: 520 | Protein: 35g | Fat: 40g | Carbs: 13g | Fiber: 3g

Ingredients:

- Six ounces Italian sausage (crumbled)
- One tbsp. oil
- One onion (chopped)
- Four ounces mushroom (sliced)
- One-fourth tsp. thyme (dried)
- One-fourth cup of each
  - Water
  - Marinara sauce
- Half tsp. oregano (dried)
- One cup cheese (shredded)
- Salt & pepper

Method:

1. Start by setting the oven temp. to 350 degrees Fahrenheit. Preheat.
2. Take a large skillet and heat oil in it over medium flame.
3. Add in the crumbled sausage to the oil and cook for about 10 mins. or until the color turns brown.
4. Cool the sausage and keep them aside.
5. Add in mushrooms and onion to the same skillet and cook until browned or for 5mins.
6. Add in the sausages to the skillet.
7. Add pepper, salt, oregano, and thyme.
8. Add water and marinara sauce to the skillet and stir well.

9. Cook the sausage for ten minutes by placing the skillet in the oven.
10. Add cheese from the top and again cook it for 5mins.
11. Serve hot.

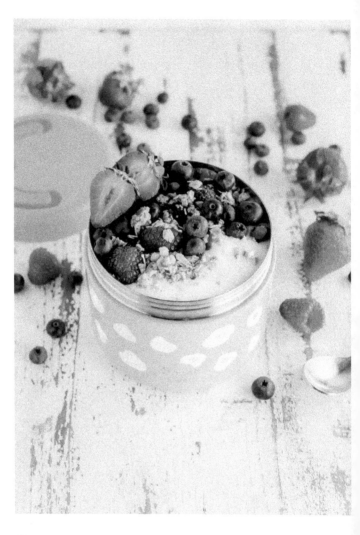

Snacks

Here are some recipes of snacks that can help you in satisfying your evening hunger with some super delicious treats.

Roasted Nuts

Total Prep & Cooking Time: 20 minutes
Yields: 4 servings
Nutrition Facts: Calories: 280 | Protein: 2g | Fat: 28g |
Carbs: 3g | Fiber: 3g

Ingredients:

- One tbsp. of olive oil
- Two cups almonds or walnuts
- One tsp. cumin (ground)
- One tsp. paprika
- Salt & pepper

Method:

1. Mix all the ingredients together in a skillet.
2. Cook for about 5 – 10 mins. until the nuts are warmed in the proper way.
3. Allow the nuts to cool for down for 5 mins.
4. Serve warm with coffee or tea.

Note: The nuts can be stored for one week in an air-tight container.

Tuna Salad Cups

Total Prep & Cooking Time: 35 minutes
Yields: 6 servings
Nutrition Facts: Calories: 250 | Protein: 19g | Fat: 2g |
Carbs: 2g | Fiber: 2g

Ingredients:

- Four bacon strips
- Four large eggs
- Two tbsps. sour cream
- One cup mayonnaise (olive oil)
- One sliced stalk of celery
- One tsp. zest of lemon
- One tbsp. fresh lemon juice
- One large tomato
- Two cans tuna (olive-oil packed)
- Two scallions (sliced)
- Sixteen lettuce leaves
- Pepper & salt

Method:

1. Take a frying pan and heat it over medium flame. Add bacon strips to the pan and cook. While cooking, crumble the cooked bacon into very small pieces.
2. Take a pot and boil water in it. Add the eggs and boil. Put the eggs in ice-cold water, peel them and roughly chop.
3. In a mixing bowl, whisk together celery, mayonnaise, sour cream, lemon juice, lemon zest, scallions, and tuna. Season with pepper and salt.

4. After mixing them well, add crumbled bacon to the bowl.
5. Cut the tomato into slices and season with pepper and salt.
6. Take one leaf of lettuce and add tomato slice for making the base. Top the tomato slices with the salad.
7. Serve hot with eggs and bacon from the top.

Cheesy Crackers

Total Prep & Cooking Time: 50 minutes
Yields: 6 servings
Nutrition Facts: Calories: 180 | Protein: 6g | Fat: 15g |
Carbs: 3g | Fiber: 3g

Ingredients:

- One cup flax meal
- One cup wheat flour or almond flour
- On cup warm water
- One cup cheese (grated)
- Two tbsps. husks (psyllium)
- Salt & pepper

Method:

1. Take a mixing bowl and mix together all the ingredients.
2. Season the mixture with pepper and salt.
3. Start adding water to the bowl and knead for making the dough.
4. Now, set your oven temp. to 350 degrees Fahrenheit. Preheat the oven.
5. Take a baking tray and place parchment paper on it. Make sure to cover the edges as well.
6. Roll out the kneaded dough on the baking tray and ensure it is thin.
7. Take a knife and cut squares in the dough.
8. Bake for about 35 minutes.

Note: The leftover crackers can be consumed later by storing it in a proper container.

Chicken Balls

Total Prep & Cooking Time: 50 minutes

Yields: 10 servings

Nutrition Facts: Calories: 280 | Protein: 13g | Fat: 25g | Carbs: 3g | Fiber: 1g

Ingredients:

- One cup shredded cheddar cheese
- Four cups chicken sausage (ground)
- One cup flour
- One cup buffalo sauce
- Three tbsps. coconut flour
- Half tsp. of each
    - Cayenne powder
    - Pepper
    - Salt

Method:

1. Start by setting the temperature of the oven to 350 degrees Fahrenheit. Preheat the oven.
2. Mix together almond flour, cheese, chicken sausage, pepper, coconut flour, salt, buffalo sauce, and cayenne powder.
3. Make small balls of one-inch size from the sausage mixture.
4. Take a baking sheet and grease it generously with cooking spray.
5. Bake the sausage balls for about half an hour or until the balls turn brown in color.

Bell Pepper Nachos

Total Prep & Cooking Time: 60 minutes
Yields: 4 servings
Nutrition Facts: Calories: 260 | Protein: 15g | Fat: 21g |
Carbs: 7g | Fiber: 5g

Ingredients:

- One tbsp. olive oil or vegetable oil
- Two large bell peppers
- One-fourth tsp. of each
  –Cumin (ground)
  –Chili powder
- One cup cheddar cheese
- Four ounces beef (ground)
- One-fourth cup guacamole
- Three tbsps. sour cream
- Half cup pico de gallo
- Salt & pepper

Also required: Broiler

Method:

1. Cut bell peppers from the stem for making medium-sized strips.
2. Take a bowl and add salt and water to it. Put in the cut bell peppers in the bowl.
3. Microwave the bell pepper for around 5 mins.
4. Take a frying pan and heat it on high flame. Add oil to the pan.
5. Add chili powder along with cumin to the pan and stir fry for around one minute.
6. Now add ground beef to the pan and add one teaspoon salt to it.

7. Continue cooking the beef until it turns brown in color.
8. Now, preheat the broiler.
9. Take one spoon of cooked beef and place them on each piece of bell pepper.
10. Add cheese from the top and broil the peppers for about 2 mins.
11. Take out the pepper and add guacamole along with pico de gallo from the top.
12. Thin the sour cream by adding water and drizzle the same over the nachos.

Note: Using pepper of different colors can provide a better presentation.

Brownie Bark

Total Prep & Cooking Time: 50 minutes
Yields: 10 servings
Nutrition Facts: Calories: 100 | Protein: 4g | Fat: 10g |
Carbs: 3g | Fiber: 1g

Ingredients:

- Two egg whites
- One cup flour (almond)
- One tsp. baking powder
- One cup butter (unsalted)
- Half cup of any sweetener
- One tsp. coffee
- Four tbsps. cocoa powder
- Half tsp. vanilla
- Half cup chocolate chips
- Two tbsp. whipping cream
- Salt

Method:

1. Start by setting the temperature of the oven to 350 degrees Fahrenheit. Preheat.
2. Take a mixing bowl and whisk in salt, almond flour, and baking powder.
3. Take a medium-sized bowl and beat the egg whites. Continue beating until it turns into a froth. Add in coffee, cocoa, and sweetener to the egg whites.
4. Add in cream, butter, and vanilla to the mixture.
5. Beat the egg mixture properly and add in flour.
6. Take a baking tray and line it properly from the edge by using a parchment paper. You can also use cooking spray.

7. Spread out the batter on the tray.
8. Bake the brownie for about half an hour.
9. Take a sharp knife and cut two-inch squares from the brownie base.
10. Warm up the brownies right before serving in the oven for about 5 mins.

Lettuce Chicken Wrap

Total Prep & Cooking Time: 15 minutes
Yields: 2 servings
Nutrition Facts: Calories: 290 | Protein: 30g | Fat: 18g |
Carbs: 3g | Fiber: 2g

Ingredients:

- One head of iceberg lettuce (remove the outer leaves and separate them from the core)
- Two bacon strips (cooked and cut in half)
- Two tbsp. mayonnaise
- One tomato (sliced)
- Three ounces of chicken breast
- Salt & pepper

Method:

1. Take a large parchment paper and spread it on your cooking area.
2. Make a layer of lettuce by placing five to seven leaves right in the middle of the paper. Try to make the base of lettuce of size 9 inches by 10 inches.
3. Take the chicken and cook it on medium flame until it turns soft. You can also shred the chicken using a spatula while cooking.
4. Spread over the mayonnaise on the lettuce base.
5. Start making a layer by using tomato, bacon, and chicken.
6. Now, start with rolling the wrap by the end which is the closest to your side. Make sure that the wrap is properly tightened, otherwise, it will open up.
7. Tuck in the end parts of the lettuce wrap from the top and bottom.

8. After completing the rolling process, keep the lettuce wrap in the refrigerator for about 30 minutes.
9. Cut the roll into half and serve cold for better taste.

Chocolate Chip Cookies

Total Prep & Cooking Time: 25 minutes
Yields: 10 servings
Nutrition Facts: Calories: 290 | Protein: 6g | Fat: 18g |
Carbs: 6g | Fiber: 2g

Ingredients:

- One cup coconut (shredded)
- Two cups flour (almond)
- One tsp. baking powder
- Half cup sweetener
- One cup of butter
- Half tsp. vanilla
- Three tsps. molasses
- One large egg
- One cup of chocolate chips
- Salt

Method:

1. Start by setting the oven temp. to 350 degrees Fahrenheit and preheat.
2. Take a mixing bowl and whisk in almond flour, coconut, baking powder, and salt.
3. Take another bowl and mix in molasses, butter, sweetener, vanilla, and egg. Add this mixture to the mixture of flour.
4. Add in chocolate chips.
5. Shape the cookie dough into small balls of half-inch size.
6. Place the balls in a baking sheet with proper gap of two inches in between.
7. Press the balls by using your hand for making them flat.
8. Bake the cookies for about 15 mins.

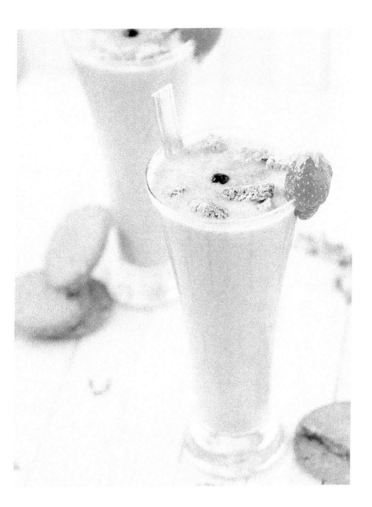

Shakes

Who doesn't love shakes, right?
While practicing intermittent fasting, your cravings
for delicious treats might increase. So, here are some
tasty recipes of shakes and smoothies that can help in
satisfying your cravings easily.

Coconut Chocolate Smoothie

Total Prep & Cooking Time: 10 minutes
Yields: 2 servings
Nutrition Facts: Calories: 510 | Protein: 26g | Fat: 37g |
Carbs: 6g | Fiber: 3g

Ingredients:

- One cup of coconut milk (full-fat, canned)
- Two tbsps. cocoa powder (unsweetened)
- Few drops of sweetener
- Ice for thickening the smoothie
- Two scoops protein (collagen)

Method:

1. Take all the ingredients except for the collagen in a food processor and blend them together. Blend them well.
2. Now, add in the collagen and blend gently for not destroying the delicate proteins.
3. Pour the smoothie in a glass.

Note: You can add extra garnishes from the top such as strawberries, apple, etc. You can also chill the smoothie in the refrigerator for about half an hour before serving. If you chill the smoothie, it will help in thickening up the consistency of the smoothie.

Cinnamon Chocolate Smoothie

Total Prep & Cooking Time: 10 minutes
Yields: 1 serving
Nutrition Facts: Calories: 290 | Protein: 4g | Fat: 32g | Carbs: 15g | Fiber: 11g

Ingredients:
- One cup of coconut milk
- Two tsps. cocoa powder (unsweetened)
- One avocado (ripe)
- One tsp. cinnamon powder
- Liquid stevia for taste
- One tsp. vanilla
- One tsp. coconut oil

Method:
1. Take all the ingredients except for stevia and blend them in a blender for about 5 mins. or until it smoothens.
2. Add in stevia according to your taste. Blend it once again for 2 mins.
3. Serve in smoothie glasses with mint leaves from the top (optional).

Note: If you want a thick smoothie, add in some ice while blending the smoothie in the blender. You can also add chocolate chips for adding texture.

Green Smoothie

Total Prep & Cooking Time: 10 minutes
Yields: 2 servings
Nutrition Facts: Calories: 150 | Protein: 3g | Fat: 12g |
Carbs: 12g | Fiber: 5g

Ingredients:
- One cup spinach
- Half cup cilantro
- One cup of water
- One peeled cucumber
- One peeled ginger
- One cup avocado (frozen)
- One peeled lemon

Method:
1. Add in all the ingredients to a blender and blend them until smooth.
2. Serve the smoothie in glasses with mint from the top.

Note: You can store the smoothie in the refrigerator for up to four days.

Avocado Mint Chocolate Smoothie

Total Prep & Cooking Time: 10 minutes
Yields: 2 servings
Nutrition Facts: Calories: 550 | Protein: 27g | Fat: 40g |
Carbs: 11g | Fiber: 8g

Ingredients:
- One cup of water
- Half cup of coconut milk
- One cup ice
- Two scoops protein powder (chocolate)
- Four mint leaves
- One cup avocado (frozen)
- One tbsp. cacao butter
- Two tbsps. coconut (shredded)

Method:
1. Put all the ingredients in the blender except for the protein powder and coconut. Blend until smooth.
2. Add in coconut and protein powder. Blend for another 20 seconds or so.
3. Serve with flakes of coconut on the top.

Note: You can use canned coconut milk.

Green Tea Cucumber Detox Smoothie

Total Prep & Cooking Time: 10 minutes
Yields: 2 servings
Nutrition Facts: Calories: 70 | Protein: 4g | Fat: 5g |
Carbs: 6g | Fiber: 3.5g

Ingredients:

- Two tsp. green tea powder
- Four cups of water
- One cucumber (sliced)
- Two cups ripe avocado (frozen)
- One tsp. fresh lemon juice
- Half tsp. liquid stevia (lemon)
- One cup ice

Method:

1. Pour in green tea powder and water in a blender. Combine both at medium speed.
2. Add in all the remaining ingredients in the blender. Blend for 5 mins. or until smooth.
3. Taste the smoothie and add liquid stevia according to your need.
4. Refrigerate the smoothie or serve immediately.

Note: You can store the smoothie in the fridge for 5 days in a proper container.

Turmeric Smoothie

Total Prep & Cooking Time: 10 minutes
Yields: 2 servings
Nutrition Facts: Calories: 550 | Protein: 6g | Fat: 57g |
Carbs: 6g | Fiber: 2g

Ingredients:

- 200 ml coconut milk (full-fat)
- 200 ml almond milk (unsweetened)
- One tbsp. turmeric powder
- One tsp. liquid sweetener
- One tsp. of each
    –Cinnamon (ground)
    –Ginger (ground)
- One tbsp. coconut oil
- One tbsp. chia seeds

Method:

1. Add all the ingredients in the blender except for the sweetener and chia seeds.
2. You can also add some ice and blend until smooth.
3. Add in liquid sweetener according to your taste.
4. Serve with chia seeds on the top.

Avocado Shake With Ginger, Turmeric, And Coconut Milk

Total Prep & Cooking Time: 25 minutes
Yields: 2 servings
Nutrition Facts: Calories: 230 | Protein: 2g | Fat: 23g |
Carbs: 6g | Fiber: 3g

Ingredients:

- One cup of coconut milk (full-fat)
- Half avocado (frozen)
- One-fourth cup almond milk
- One tsp. turmeric powder
- One tsp. fresh lemon juice
- Liquid sweetener (sugar-free)
- One cup ice
- One tsp. ginger (grated)

Method:

1. Add in all the ingredients in the blender except for ice and sweetener.
2. Blend until smooth.
3. Add in sweetener according to your taste. Blend for a few seconds.
4. Pour ice in the blender and blend in high speed for 2 – 3 mins.
5. Serve immediately or store in the refrigerator for later consumption.

Note: You can a pinch of black pepper in the smoothie for improving the taste.

Marshmallow Vanilla Smoothie

Total Prep & Cooking Time: 10 minutes
Yields: 2 servings
Nutrition Facts: Calories: 290 | Protein: 6g | Fat: 18g |
Carbs: 6g | Fiber: 2g

Ingredients:

- Three cups ice
- One cup of water
- One cup marshmallow (any flavor)
- One cup of coconut milk (full-fat)
- Two tbsps. chia seeds or flax seeds
- Two tbsps. protein powder
- One tsp. gluten-free vanilla extract
- Honey or liquid stevia for sweetness

Method:

1. Add all the ingredients in the blender except for ice and honey.
2. Blend until the marshmallow gets mixed properly.
3. Add in honey according to your taste. Blend for mixing it in.
4. Put ice in the blender and blend for thickening up the smoothie.
5. Serve with shredded coconut from the top (optional).

Note: You can also use canned coconut milk. Also, the smoothie can be stored in the fridge for two days.

Conclusion

Thank you for making it through to the end of Intermittent Fasting For Women Over 50: The Easier Guide to Master The Secrets of Losing Weight. Detoxify The Body and Gain Energy to Promote Longevity!
I hope it was informative overall and was capable of delivering you with all the information that you needed to achieve all your goals.

You are now required to start applying all that you have just learned from this book in your everyday life. Do not try to delay it as the perfect day is never going to come. The perfect time for beginning with something brand new is now. The world of diet is changing every day and it might also turn out to be very tiresome for you to cope up with all the trends, that too with growing age. As you start with the process of intermittent fasting, you will soon be realizing that nothing else is needed. Intermittent fasting alone can easily deal with all your problems. You just need to ensure that you perform it in the proper way.

The main benefit of intermittent fasting is that you will no longer need to count all the calories that you consume. Intermittent fasting is all about maintaining a healthy body and life by fasting at specific intervals of time. You can carry on with your normal diet for the rest of the time. You can choose from the wide variety of choices available for you for intermittent fasting.

If you find this book helpful for yourself in any way, kindly leave a review.

CPSIA information can be obtained
at www.ICGtesting.com
Printed in the USA
BVHW041725230221
600894BV00015B/1763